2004

PCAT SUCCESS

MW00906958

Dick R. Gourley, B.S. Ph., Pharm.D.
Greta A. Gourley, B.S.N., M.S.N., Pharm.D., Ph.D.

TEST PREP

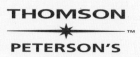
THOMSON

PETERSON'S

Australia • Canada • Mexico • Singapore • Spain • United Kingdom • United States

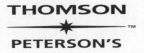

About The Thomson Corporation and Peterson's

With revenues of US$7.8 billion, The Thomson Corporation (www.thomson.com) is a leading global provider of integrated information solutions for business, education, and professional customers. Its Learning businesses and brands (www.thomsonlearning.com) serve the needs of individuals, learning institutions, and corporations with products and services for both traditional and distributed learning.

Peterson's, part of The Thomson Corporation, is one of the nation's most respected providers of lifelong learning online resources, software, reference guides, and books. The Education Supersite[sm] at www.petersons.com—the Internet's most heavily traveled education resource—has searchable databases and interactive tools for contacting U.S.-accredited institutions and programs. In addition, Peterson's serves more than 105 million education consumers annually.

For more information, contact Peterson's, 2000 Lenox Drive, Lawrenceville, NJ 08648; 800-338-3282; or find us on the World Wide Web at: www.petersons.com/about.

COPYRIGHT © 2004 Peterson's, a division of Thomson Learning, Inc. Thomson Learning™ is a trademark used herein under license.

Previous editions © 1984, 1991, 1997, 2000, 2001, 2002

ALL RIGHTS RESERVED. No part of this work covered by the copyright herein may be reproduced or used in any form or by any means—graphic, electronic, or mechanical, including photocopying, recording, taping, Web distribution, or information storage and retrieval systems—without the prior written permission of the publisher.

For permission to use material from this text or product, contact us by
Phone: 800-730-2214
Fax: 800-730-2215
Web: www.thomsonrights.com

ISBN: 0-7689-1309-8

Printed in the United States of America

10 9 8 7 6 5 4 3 2 1   05 04 03

Contributing Editors

Verbal Ability Section

Greta A. Gourley, B.S.N., M.S.N., Pharm.D, Ph.D.
Associate Professor of Pharmaceutical Sciences
College of Pharmacy
University of Tennessee Health Science Center, Memphis, TN

Biology Section

Ryan Yates, Pharm.D., Ph.D.
Assistant Professor of Pharmaceutical Sciences
College of Pharmacy
University of Tennessee Health Science Center, Memphis, TN

Quantitative Ability Section

George Bass, Ph.D.
Associate Professor of Pharmaceutical Sciences
University of Tennessee Health Science Center, Memphis, TN

Arthur B. Straughn, B.S.Ph., Pharm.D.
Professor of Pharmaceutical Sciences
College of Pharmacy
University of Tennessee Health Science Center, Memphis, TN

Chemistry Section

Wi Lei, M.Sc., Ph.D.
Instructor Pharmaceutical Sciences
University of Tennessee Health Science Center, Memphis, TN

Duane D. Miller, B.S.Ph., M.S., Ph.D.
Van Vleet Professor of Pharmaceutical Sciences and Associate Dean for Research and Graduate Affairs
College of Pharmacy
University of Tennessee Health Science Center, Memphis, TN

Reading Comprehension Section

Dick R. Gourley, B.S.Ph., Pharm.D.
Professor of Pharmacy and Dean of College of Pharmacy
University of Tennessee Health Science Center, Memphis, TN

Contents

Introduction to Pharmacy Practice

HISTORICAL PERSPECTIVE

The pharmacy profession can be traced to approximately 3000 B.C.E.—the time of ancient Babylonia-Assyria, Egypt, and Greece. Although very little is known of pharmacy at that time, fragments of knowledge remain. The word *pharmacy* and its derivatives can be traced this far back and to some degree, explain the meaning of the Greek word *pharmakon*. Opinions are divided as to whether pharmacists existed in ancient Egypt, or if they were actually "physician assistants" who specialized in the preparation of pharmaceuticals.

Pharmacy was originally the work of priests. Later it became part of the function of lay medical practitioners, who combined medicine and pharmacy. The birth of European professional pharmacy occurred around 1240 C.E., when the German Emperor Frederick II issued "an edict that was to be the Magna Charta of the profession of pharmacy" (see Kramer and Urdang's *History of Pharmacy*, Lippincott, Philadelphia, 1963). As the practices of pharmacy grew and matured, pharmacists became responsible for preparing and dispensing medications, and in European societies, became known as the apothecary. At the same time, the physician became responsible for diagnosing and treating illness.

The profession of pharmacy evolved from an apprenticeship, requiring no formal education, to a sophisticated professional degree program. At the turn of the eighteenth century, pharmacy education was approximately 10 percent education and 90 percent practice.

The Philadelphia School of Pharmacy and Sciences, founded in 1821, was the first school of pharmacy in the United States. The first state university—Medical College of South Carolina—was founded in 1867. The early schools of pharmacy were privately owned and were used to educate physicians as well as pharmacists.

The standard dictionary definition of *pharmacy* is "the art or practice of preparing, preserving, compounding, and dispensing drugs." These were the traditional roles of the pharmacist. However, career opportunities in pharmacy are much broader today and include, but are not limited to, the following:

- Storing and purchasing medications
- Advising patients and other health-care providers on medications
- Provision of Drug Information Services to health-care providers
- Manufacturing/Quality Control
- Pharmaceutical Sales
- Education
- Practice, research, and administration with various government agencies, health-care institutions, and community pharmacies
- Development of health policy
- Specialty pharmacy practice (e.g. geriatrics, pediatrics, oncology, or nuclear pharmacy)

Technology has made a dramatic difference in the provision of health care. Likewise, the role of the pharmacist as health-care professional has expanded with the development of the pharmaceutical care movement.

PATIENT-CENTERED PHARMACEUTICAL CARE ERA

During the early part of the twentieth century, pharmacists compounded medications and practiced primarily in the corner drug store. In the 1940s and 1950s, the pharmaceutical industry began to expand rapidly and manufacture medications that had to be dispensed. There was still compounding, but from the 1940s to the 1960s, pharmacist compounding diminished. Then in the 1960s, the clinical movement in pharmacy began, which eventually led to pharmaceutical care.

Since the 1960s, pharmacy has moved from a product-oriented profession toward a more patient-oriented practice. This shift is a result of the increase in new drug products on the market, and consequently, the greater need for patient information and education about those drugs, as well as the increased cost of health care.

Likewise, pharmacy education has moved from a chemistry/laboratory-based education to a more biological/practice-based education. Automation and technology continue to expand the pharmacist's role from a dispenser of medications to a patient education specialist—called upon to resolve therapeutic dilemmas and provide patient education.

Pharmaceutical care was first defined by Mikeal, et al in 1975, as "the care that a given patient requires and receives which assures safe and rational drug usage." In 1980, Donald C. Brodie suggested that pharmaceutical care includes the determination of the drug needs for a patient and includes the concept of a feedback mechanism to facilitate continuity of care.

Charles D. Hepler described pharmaceutical care as "a covenantal relationship between a patient and a pharmacist in which the pharmacist performs drug-use-control functions (with appropriate knowledge and skill) governed by awareness of a commitment to the patient's interest." Hepler and L.M. Strand indicated that "pharmaceutical care is the responsible provision of drug therapy for the purpose of achieving a definite outcome that improves a patient's quality of life."

J.A. Johnson and J.L. Bootman reported in 1995, that, as a result of drug-related illnesses, ambulatory patients in the United States spend more than $76 billion annually—a sum exceeding the cost of the drug therapy itself. This estimate does not include the indirect costs of drug-related illnesses, such as loss of work and productivity. Pharmacists are positioned to play a major role in improving patient compliance/adherence to drug therapy regimens and to resolving this $76 billion problem. Since the Johnson and Bootman study, recent estimates conclude that the costs of drug-related illnesses are in excess of $100 billion per year. Managed care demands an increased level of pharmacist involvement in patient care to improve health care as well as to control costs. Likewise, patients have become more assertive in their quest for information about medications and diseases. Direct-to-consumer advertising has increased the level of patient knowledge and heightened the awareness of the need for information.

Pharmacist Responsibilities for Patient-Centered Pharmaceutical Care

1. **Patient Education**—Discuss the correct way for patients to take medication; educate patients about disease; and answer questions about drug therapy, drug interactions, and issues such as diet and exercise.

2. **Monitoring**—Monitor patients' therapy to assure that their medications are working effectively, with no side effects or adverse drug reactions (ADR). Assess patients' understanding of disease and drug therapy in order to improve patient compliance/adherence.

3. **Providing pharmacokinetic consultations**—Provide information to physicians on drug absorption, drug excretion, and drug metabolism of specific drugs, allowing for individualized dosing and assuring optimal drug therapy results.

4. **Relating drug information**—Provide information to physicians, nurses, dentists, and other health-care providers as well as to the public.

5. **Prescribing**—Pharmacists have traditionally been responsible for recommending over-the-counter drugs to patients. However, over the past several years there have been changes in pharmacy practice laws in several states. These changes provide for pharmacists prescribing under protocol, and also for collaborative-care agreements between pharmacists and physicians as well as other health-care providers.

6. **Disease Management**—Work in concert with other health-care professionals to provide disease management for specific patient populations. For example, diabetes and asthma are two chronic diseases with which pharmacists have been actively involved as members of the disease management team.

A recent Gallup Poll recognized pharmacists as one of the five most trusted professionals for the tenth year in a row. (Darren K. Carlson. Nurses Remain at Top of Honesty and Ethics Poll. *Gallup Poll News Service.* November 27, 2000). Because of their relationship with, and availability to, the public, pharmacists are uniquely positioned to assume these expanded roles.

If you want to read more about the pharmacist's responsibilities in patient-centered pharmaceutical care, we recommend the following references:

1. "Standards of Practice for the Profession of Pharmacy," *American Pharmacy* 19, no. 3 (1979): 31.

2. "Pharmacy in the 21st Century Conference: Executive Summary," *The Consultant Pharmacist* 5, no. 4 (April 1990): 226-233.

3. Manasse, Henri R. Jr. "Medication Use in an Imperfect World," American Society of Hospital Pharmacists, 1989; 46:929-44 and 1989; 46:1141-52.

4. Hepler, C. D. The third wave in pharmaceutical education: the clinical movement. *Am. J. Pharm. Ed.* 1987; 51:369-384.

5. Cocolas, G. H. Pharmacy in the 21st century conference: executive summary. *Am. J. Pharm. Ed.* Winter. 1989;53(WS): 15-55.

6. Brodie, D. C., Parish, P.A., and Poston, J.W. Social needs for drugs and drug-related services. *Am J Pharm Ed.* 1987; 51:369-85.

7. Proceedings: Understanding and preventing drug misadventures. A multidisciplinary invitational conference sponsored by the ASHP Research and Education Foundation in cooperation with the American Medical Association, the American Nurses Association, and the American Society of Hospital Pharmacists. *Am J Health-Syst Pharm.* 1995; 52:369–416.

8. Gourley D. R. Curriculum evolution: What progress have we made? *Am J Pharm Ed.* 1989; 53:375-9.

A study of the future of pharmacy practice and education, *Pharmacists for the Future,* was conducted and published in 1975. It provides an in-depth analysis of past and present trends in the pharmacy profession and discusses the roles that future pharmacists will fulfill. The following quotation is from the Millis Commission report, *Pharmacists for the Future,* the Report of the Study Commission on Pharmacy. Health Administration Press, Ann Arbor, 1975:

> Pharmacy should be defined basically as a system, which renders a health service by concerning itself with knowledge about drugs and their effects upon man and animal. Pharmacy generates knowledge about drugs, acquires relevant knowledge from the biological, chemical, physical, and behavioral sciences; it tests, organizes, and applies that knowledge. Pharmacy translates a substantial portion of that knowledge into drug products and distributes them widely to those who require them. Pharmacy knowledge is disseminated to physicians, pharmacists, other health-care providers, and to the general public to the end that drug knowledge and products may contribute to the health of individuals and to the welfare of society. The knowledge system of pharmacy through its therapeutic use is a substantial and significant segment of health care in the United States.

FACTORS AFFECTING THE PHARMACY PROFESSION

There are both internal and external factors to the pharmacy profession that affect the future of the pharmacy profession. The following comments address six factors that have made an impact on the pharmacy profession. Further information can be found in each of these areas by consulting publications relevant in pharmacy literature.

1. **Federal Legislation:** Federal legislation, such as the Health Information Privacy Protection Act (HIPPA), has had a significant impact on the functioning of all health-care professionals, including pharmacists. HIPPA primarily affects the record-keeping systems in pharmacy and the patient's right to privacy. Other legislation, such as the prescription drug benefit for Medicare patients, also has a major impact on the pharmacy profession.

2. **Aging U.S. Population:** As a greater percentage of U.S. citizens exceed 65 years of age, the demand for pharmacy services will grow as the number of prescriptions dispensed will increase. In 2002, approximately 2.2 billion prescriptions were dispensed. By 2004, it is projected is that more than 4.4 billion prescriptions will be dispensed, creating a continuing demand for pharmacists.

3. **Corporate Mergers:** Corporate mergers have an effect on the pharmaceutical industry, as well as the hospital and chain drug industries.

4. **Automation/Technology:** As automation and technology advance, the pharmacist's ability to provide better patient care will be enhanced.

5. **Drug Development:** New medications mean the ability to treat patients more effectively and the need for pharmacists to provide new drug information to patients and health-care providers.

6. **Staffing:** There is a shortage of pharmacists, nurses, allied health professionals, and, in some locations, dentists and medical specialists. Due to this shortage, the starting salaries of pharmacists have increased dramatically over the past four years. In 2002, the average starting salary for graduates in the Southeast was in excess of $80,000.

CAREER OPPORTUNITIES

Since the 1960s, pharmacy education and practice have undergone incredible changes—changes that continue into the twenty-first century. Pharmacy, an old and honored profession, is still evolving. Job opportunities are available in a variety of areas, including, but not limited to the following:

- Community pharmacy (independent practice or chain store)
- Hospital pharmacy
- Pharmaceutical industry
- Government
- Geriatric pharmacy
- Pediatrics and other clinical practice areas
- Veterinary pharmacy
- Compounding
- Home infusion

Current job opportunities also include clinical practice in a variety of specialty areas, including nuclear pharmacy, pharmacotherapy, nutrition support practice, psychiatric practice, and oncology practice. These areas are recognized by the Board of Pharmaceutical Specialties. In addition, practice in managed care is still evolving, and there will be opportunities in areas not yet identified.

Educational opportunities beyond the pharmacy degree include graduate education in the pharmaceutical or medical sciences, including medicine and dentistry. The opportunity to further your education in a collateral area by combining a pharmacy career with a law degree or MBA, for example, exists as well.

Individuals who complete either a Bachelor of Science in pharmacy (B.S.) or a Doctor of Pharmacy degree (Pharm.D.) have many opportunities available to them. Postgraduate education also offers an excellent opportunity for building upon the basic pharmacy education.

Note: The American Council On Pharmaceutical Education (ACPE) announced in July of 1997 that the Pharm.D. would be the only accredited entry-level degree in pharmacy. All colleges of pharmacy in the United States now offer the Pharm.D. as the entry-level professional degree.

The following are brief descriptions of some of the career opportunities available when the basic requirements for pharmacy licensure are completed.

Community/Ambulatory Practice

Community pharmacists are becoming practitioners who provide a variety of health-care services to patients, including: dispensing medications; providing patient education on disease and medications; and performing immunizations, allergy shots, and therapeutic drug monitoring. In addition to these responsibilities, pharmacists are also responsible for educating the patient about their medications.

Because of the ever-increasing quantity of pharmaceutical knowledge, professionals in other areas of health care turn more frequently to pharmacists for advice and assistance. For instance, pharmacists may contribute information on selecting the best drug therapy for a patient and help physicians monitor a patient's progress. Pharmacists must detect possible adverse reactions as a result of drug-drug, drug-food, and drug-disease interactions. They also have the responsibility of advising patients in the use of nonprescription drugs. In addition, they must make recommendations to patients and other health professionals for avoiding problems with drug use.

The practice of community pharmacy is also a business. In addition to patient-care activities, pharmacists must also manage people, resources, and time. The opportunity for community involvement and the respect of the patient make community practice exciting. Opportunities are available in rural and metropolitan areas as well as in a variety of settings, such as apothecaries, chain stores, and independent community pharmacies.

For more information about community/ambulatory practice, contact the American Pharmaceutical Association (APhA), 2215 Constitution Avenue NW, Washington, D.C. 20037-2985; phone: (202) 628-4410 or fax: (202) 783-2351; Web site: www.aphanet.org.

Institutional Pharmacy

Pharmacists in institutions supervise the distribution of drugs to patients, provide therapeutic drug monitoring, formulary services, drug information services, and management services. In addition, pharmacists are assuming greater responsibility for patient education. This includes taking medication histories of admitted patients, monitoring drug therapies, managing the drug regimens of patients, and making patient rounds with physicians and nurses to provide drug information, participate in cardiac codes, and provide pharmacokinetic and therapeutic consultations to physicians, physician's assistants, and advanced practice nurses.

Pharmacists serve as consultants to other health professionals on drug therapy and conduct in-service education programs for them. In addition, some pharmacists may work in a nuclear pharmacy, preparing various radioactive testing agents as well as radio pharmaceuticals used in chemotherapy regimens for cancer patients.

Decentralization of pharmacy services expanded institutional pharmacy to a more clinical role. Institutional pharmacists specialize in a variety of areas, including practice management, critical care, ambulatory care, geriatrics, pediatrics, medicine, surgery, oncology, psychiatry, nutrition support, and drug education. Clinical practice changed the role of the pharmacist to that of a provider of pharmaceutical care.

For more information about institutional pharmacy practice contact the American Society of Health-Systems Pharmacists (ASHP), 7272 Wisconsin Avenue, Bethesda, MD 20814; phone: (301) 657-3000 or fax: (301) 652-8278; Web site: www.ashp.org.

Pharmaceutical Industry

Many pharmaceutical firms employ pharmacists in clinical research, product development, quality control, sales, marketing, management, and several other roles. Pharmacists, as well as other scientists, are responsible for testing and controlling the production of drugs. Once pharmaceuticals have been manufactured, they must be marketed. Pharmacists work in regulatory affairs, dealing with the Food and Drug Administration (FDA), as well as in professional affairs. The professional affairs area includes working with other pharmacists, physicians, and health-care providers, as well as with the general public.

Pharmacists also serve as medical service representatives—the sales force of the pharmaceutical industry. These representatives call on physicians, dentists, veterinarians, pharmacists (hospital, community, extended care facilities, and government agencies) and nurses to explain the uses and merits of the products that their firms manufacture. In addition, the clinical research area uses pharmacists to monitor and control field research and to select research sites.

Another area of the pharmaceutical industry is product and consumer information. Pharmacists in this part of the field provide product information to health care providers and to the public. They also serve as a resource for sales and marketing forces. For more information on opportunities in the pharmaceutical industry, contact The Pharmaceutical Research and Manufacturers of America (PhRMA); 1100 15th Street NW, Suite 800, Washington, D.C. 20005; phone: (202) 835-3400 or fax: (202) 835-3414; Web site: www.phrma.org.

Government Pharmacy Practice

Many pharmacists work for public health departments on a federal, state, or local level. In the FDA, pharmacists work with physicians and other health-care providers in assessing sound manufacturing practices and the efficacy of new drug products. In the U.S. Public Health Service, pharmacists are employed as institutional pharmacy practitioners, administrators, or clinical pharmacists. Pharmacy positions are also available in other government agencies, such as the National Institutes of Health, where practitioners provide patient-centered pharmaceutical care and also conduct research.

Pharmacists may participate at the local or state government level as members of licensing boards (State Boards of Pharmacy) as administrators, inspectors, or board members. Pharmaceutical services are also provided in health-care facilities on military bases in the United States and abroad. Each branch of the armed forces has pharmacists that are commissioned officers.

For further information on career opportunities in the federal government contact the appropriate agency from the following:

U.S. Department of Veterans Affairs; 810 Vermont Avenue NW; Washington, D.C. 20420; phone: (202) 273-8426; fax: (202) 273-9067; e-mail: ogden.john@mail.va.gov

U.S. Air Force; 89th Medical Group; 1050 West Perimeter; Suite D1-119; Andrews AFB, MD 20762-6600; phone: (301) 981-2848; fax: (301) 981-4544

U.S. Army; Walter Reed Army Medical Center; Washington, D.C. 20307-5001; phone: (202) 782-6072; fax: (202) 782-0410; e-mail: kent.maneval@na.amedd.army.mil

U.S. Navy; National Naval Medical Center; Bethesda, MD 20889-5600; phone: (301) 295-2120; fax: (301) 295-4662

U.S. Public Health Service (USPHS); 5600 Fishers Lane, Room 9A-05; Rockville, MD 20857; phone: (301) 443-7773; fax: (301) 549-1171; e-mail: fpaavola@hrsa.ss

Nuclear Pharmacy

Nuclear pharmacy is a unique specialty area within pharmacy. Individuals who specialize in nuclear pharmacy work with and prepare radioactive medications (diagnostic or therapeutic agents). Pharmacists must be certified to work with radioactive materials; generally a postgraduate course is required. Pharmacy students may take electives in nuclear pharmacy in schools of pharmacy that offer such programs. Postgraduate courses may cover the minimum requirement of 200 hours of work or may include graduate course work leading to an M.S. degree or Ph.D. Nuclear Pharmacy was the first board-certified specialty recognized by the Board of Pharmaceutical Specialties.

For more information on nuclear pharmacy and other pharmacy specialties contact: Board of Pharmaceutical Specialties (BPS), 2215 Constitution Avenue NW, Washington, D.C. 20037-2985; phone: (202) 429-7591 or fax: (202) 783-2351.

Geriatric Pharmacy Practice

The fastest growing segment of the population consists of individuals over the age of 65. In 1880, this group represented 3 percent of the population, while in 1980 it represented 11.3 percent of the population. It is estimated that by the year 2010, 22.5 percent of the population will be over the age 65.

Geriatric patients have more chronic diseases and therefore use more over-the-counter prescription medications than any other age group. Because of their medication needs and the unique problems of drug therapy for the elderly, a specialty in geriatric pharmacy practice developed. This practitioner provides therapeutic consultation, patient counseling and education, in-service education to nursing staffs of extended-care facilities, and therapeutic consultations with physicians on the drug therapy regimens of the elderly. In addition, dispensing services are also required for these facilities. This new area of practice offers a rewarding and challenging career.

For more information on geriatric pharmacy or consultant practice contact: American Society of Consultant Pharmacists, 1321 Duke Street, Alexandria, VA 22314-3563; phone: (703) 739-1300 or fax: (703) 739-1321; Web site: www.ascp.com.

Clinical Practice Specialty Areas

During the past twenty years, a clinical practice of pharmacy developed that focused on the provision of rational therapeutics to patients in specific areas. For example, there are pharmacists who now practice in specialty areas such as pediatrics, oncology, psychiatry, critical-care medicine, pharmacokinetics, geriatrics, pulmonary medicine, and infectious diseases. These practitioners provide services to patients in hospitals and/or clinic situations.

In the future, a residency or fellowship will be required in addition to the basic Pharm.D. degree in order to practice in specialty areas. The majority of these practitioners today have a Pharm.D. degree and either a specialty residency or fellowship. Specialties that are recognized for board certification by the Board of Pharmaceutical Specialties include nutrition support pharmacy, pharmacotherapy, psychiatry pharmacy practice, and oncology pharmacy practice.

For more information on board certification of pharmacists contact: Board of Pharmaceutical Specialties (BPS), 2215 Constitution Avenue NW, Washington, D.C. 20037-2985; phone: (202) 429-7591 or fax: (202) 783-2351.

For more information on specialty clinical practice areas in pharmacy contact: American College of Clinical Pharmacy (ACCP); 3101 Broadway, Suite 380; Kansas City, MO 64111; phone: (816) 531-2177 or fax: (816) 531-4990; Web site: www.accp.com.

* * *

The pharmacy profession is dynamic and ever-changing. If you select pharmacy as your career goal, you will find it rewarding and challenging. Contact a college/school of pharmacy or your state pharmacy association for more information on pharmacy career opportunities and pharmacy education.

PART I

Preparing for Your Pharmacy Career

Chapter 1: Pharmacy Education

ACCREDITATION OF PHARMACY EDUCATION

Pharmacy colleges are accredited by the American Council on Pharmaceutical Education (ACPE). The ACPE was established in 1932 and is the national accrediting agency in pharmacy recognized by the Secretary of Education, U.S. Department of Education, and the Council on Post-Secondary Accreditation (COPA). The ACPE is also a member of the Council of Specialized Accrediting Agencies.

The ACPE is an autonomous agency whose membership is derived through the American Association of Colleges of Pharmacy (AACP), the American Pharmaceutical Association (APhA), and the National Association of Boards of Pharmacy (NABP), with three members appointed by each of the respective associations. In addition, there is one member appointed from the American Council on Education (ACE), making ten council members. Also, a panel of public representatives serves in an advisory capacity to the council and provides for public contribution to its proceedings. The American Foundation for Pharmaceutical Education provides major financial support for the council's general activities. The AACP, APhA, and NABP also provide annual support to sustain the council's activities. Colleges pay an annual fee to the ACPE to sustain their accreditation status and also pay for related expenses when accredited.

A list of accredited degree programs is published annually by the ACPE and is available upon request. Contact the American Council on Pharmaceutical Education (ACPE), One East Wacker Drive, Chicago, IL 60601; phone: (312) 664-3575 or fax: (312) 664-4652; Web site: www.acpe-accredit.org.

You must graduate from a college or school of pharmacy that is accredited by the American Council on Pharmaceutical Education to be eligible to take the NABPLEX examination given by the state board of pharmacy in your state. Each state gives the examination with the exception of California, which conducts its own examination. You should contact your state to determine how the board examination is given, and any other questions concerning state requirements.

For more information contact the National Association of Boards of Pharmacy (NABP), 700 Busse Highway, Park Ridge, IL 60068-2402; phone: (847) 698-6227 or fax: (847) 698-0124; e-mail: ceo@napb.net; Web site: www.napb.net.

INSTITUTIONS AND PROGRAMS

As of this printing, there are eighty-five U.S. colleges and schools of pharmacy. Seventy-seven have accredited first professional degree programs, and four have programs in pre-candidate accreditation status. Contact the individual school of pharmacy for information on a specific school's accreditation status.

Twenty-six programs are in private institutions while fifty-five are in publicly-supported universities. There are three independent, free-standing pharmacy schools, all private. The remaining seventy-eight schools are university affiliated. Thirty-five schools of pharmacy are part of an academic health center campus.

While each college of pharmacy curriculum has the same basic courses, the variation occurs in the course sequence, credit hours per courses, elective courses, total number of hours required for graduation, and pre-pharmacy requirements.

At the American Association of Colleges of Pharmacy (AACP) annual meeting in July 1992, pharmacy faculty members voted to move toward the Pharm.D. as the only entry-level professional degree in pharmacy. In July of 1997, the American Council on Pharmaceutical Education (ACPE) adopted new accreditation standards and guidelines that, resulted in accreditation only for colleges or schools who offer the Pharm.D. Today, all schools of pharmacy have implemented the Pharm.D. degree as the entry-level degree.

PHARMACY STUDENTS

Pharmacy student enrollment ranged from 52 to 1,482 students per school in 2001–02. Schools reported an application to enrollment ratio of approximately 2.9:1. The AACP's annual Applicant Pool Survey indicated that, from September 2000 through August 2001, eighty-two schools and colleges received 26,265 applications to first professional degree programs—a 9.1 percent increase from the previous year. According to the survey, 66.3 percent of the applications were from women and 33.7 percent were from men. Applications from African Americans represented 10.8 percent of the total applications for 2000–01; applications from the Hispanic population, 4 percent; and applications from Native Americans, 0.5 percent. Of the applicants in 2000–01, 55.3 percent were submitted by students who had completed three or more years of postsecondary education; 29 percent had completed three or more years without earning a degree; 25.2 percent held a baccalaureate; 0.9 percent held a master's degree; and 0.2 percent held a doctorate.

The total full-time pharmacy professional student enrollment in first professional degree programs was 35,885 in the Fall of 2001. Of these, 2,978 were enrolled in B.S. programs and 32,907 in Pharm.D. degree programs. More than 64 percent of the total students were women and more than 12 percent were minority students: African American (8.8 percent), Hispanic (5.3 percent) and Native American (less than 1 percent).

Total full-time graduate student enrollment in 2001 was 3,084: 2,264 students in Ph.D. and 820 in M.S. programs. 51 percent of full-time graduate students in the M.S. programs were female and 49 percent were male. In Ph.D. programs, 53.1 percent were male and 46.9 percent were female.

The total number of professional degrees conferred in 2001 was 7,000—a decrease of 3.6 percent from 1999–2000. Women received 64.5 percent of the first professional degrees and men received 35.5 percent. Of the first professional degrees conferred, 27.3 percent were B.S. and 72.7 percent were Pharm.D. The total number of M.S. degrees conferred was 461 (an increase of 23.2 percent from 1999–2000). There were 375 Ph.D. degrees awarded (an increase of 16.1 percent from 1999–2000).

Note: Above data were compiled from the AACP Profile of Students Report, Fall, 2001.

COMPONENTS OF PHARMACY EDUCATION

Pharmacy education can be divided into five distinct components:

1. **Pre-pharmacy education,** which requires two years as a minimum and may be taken at a junior college, community college, four-year college, or a university. (Time may be reduced by taking an accelerated load, although this is not necessarily recommended.) Approximately 24 percent of students entering pharmacy in 1999 held a B.S. degree, and many students had three years of pre-pharmacy education.

2. **Professional pharmacy education,** which takes either three years (year-round Pharm.D. degree) or four years (Pharm.D. degree), and must be taken at one of the eighty-one accredited schools or colleges of pharmacy in the United States in order to qualify to take the NABPLEX examination for licensure.

3. **Graduate education,** which leads to a M.S. or Ph.D. degree.

4. **Residency or fellowship programs** following either the B.S. or Pharm.D. entry-level degree. These are one- or two-year professional experiences, offered in a variety of practice settings.

5. **Professional continuing pharmaceutical education,** which is a requirement for continued licensure as a pharmacist. Each state board of pharmacy has state-specific requirements. The majority of states require that pharmacists obtain 15 contact hours (1.5 C.E.U.) each year to maintain their licenses.

DEGREES OFFERED

There are two professional pharmacy degrees offered by schools and colleges of pharmacy as the entry-level degree:

1. The Bachelor of Science in Pharmacy—B.S. (*Note*: This will be phased out by 2004.)
2. The Doctor of Pharmacy—Pharm.D.

The graduate degrees offered in the pharmaceutical sciences include the following:

1. Master of Science—M.S.
2. Doctor of Philosophy—Ph.D.

Fifty-six pharmacy colleges offer graduate programs. Graduate programs at the master's and doctoral levels include the focus areas of medicinal chemistry, pharmaceuticals, pharmacology, toxicology, pharmacokinetics, drug metabolism, molecular modeling, and nuclear pharmacy. This list is not all-inclusive. Many colleges also offer the Ph.D. and master's degree in health science administration, pharmacoeconomics, and pharmacy administration.

There are several colleges of pharmacy that offer a joint Pharm.D./Ph.D. program. In these programs, students take all of their electives in the graduate school and must have either a previous B.S. degree in an area other than pharmacy or three years of pre-pharmacy with significant course work beyond the pre-pharmacy requirements in order to enter the program.

Another very popular combined graduate program is the joint B.S./MBA or Pharm.D./MBA. As of this printing, these programs are offered by thirteen colleges of pharmacy in conjunction with a school of business. Students with the joint degree are very attractive job candidates to the government, the pharmaceutical industry, and the chain drug industry.

For information on graduate education programs and on joint undergraduate professional and graduate degree programs, contact the school or college of pharmacy that you are considering. You should also inquire about how many graduates enter residencies or fellowships following graduation.

PRE-PHARMACY REQUIREMENTS

Most pharmacy schools or colleges require two years of pre-pharmacy for entrance into the professional curriculum. Some programs have a 0-6 (pre-pharmacy/professional) program while others have a 1-5, 2-4, or a 3-4 program. A two-year pre-pharmacy curriculum includes either 60-semester hours or 90-quarter hours, depending upon the particular program. The following minimum requirements for admission are for the University of Tennessee College of Pharmacy (UT) and are provided for guidance only. Requirements for colleges of pharmacy vary; the major difference is in the number of required hours in physics, organic chemistry, and mathematics. Students should contact each institution for specific information about requirements.

UT's minimum requirements for admission to its College of Pharmacy are as follows:

1. Completion of 66-semester hours with 50-semester hours of required pre-pharmacy courses and 16-semester hours of elective courses.

2. PCAT is required at UT (See lists of colleges and schools for those that require the PCAT). A composite scaled score of 190 is required; however, this score is not a competitive score.

3. A personal interview and three letters of reference are required.

4. A grade of C or above must be obtained in each required course.

Pre-pharmacy Curriculum for Fall 2003
University of Tennessee College of Pharmacy

Course Semester	Hours
General Chemistry	8
Organic Chemistry	8
General Biology/Zoology	8
Physics	8
Microbiology	3
English Composition	6
Communications/Speech (Interpersonal skills, not drama or theater)	3
Statistics	3
Fundamentals of Calculus	3
Social Science Electives (Psychology, Sociology, Economics, Anthropology, Political Science)	6
Humanities Electives (Literature, Language, History, Philosophy)	6
General Electives	4
TOTAL	**66***

Note: One year of American History (high school or college level) is required for graduation from the University of Tennessee.

*The total pre-pharmacy hours will increase from 66 to 90 hours for the class entering in the fall of 2005.

For information on pre-pharmacy requirements, graduate education programs, joint undergraduate professional, and graduate degree programs, contact the college or school of pharmacy that you are considering. Also, note that a few colleges of pharmacy now require a B.S. degree or three years of pre-pharmacy to enter the Pharm.D. professional degree program.

PROFESSIONAL PHARMACY CURRICULUM

The pharmacy curriculum is comprised of basic science and clinical science courses. The following is an example of a Pharm.D. curriculum for the University of Tennessee. This curriculum provides an example of the intensity and content of the pharmacy curriculum.

Doctor of Pharmacy Curriculum
(University of Tennessee)

FIRST PROFESSIONAL YEAR

Fall Semester	Semester Hours	Lecture/Laboratory
ANAT 111 Anatomy	3	(2/2)
BIOC 111 Biochemistry	5	(4/2)
PHSC 112 Medicinal Chemistry I	3	(3/0)
PPE 132 Intro. Pharmacy & the Health-Care Environment	3	(2/2)
PHSC 111 Physical Pharmacy	3	(3/0)
PHSC 113 Pharmacy Math	1	(1/0)
TOTAL HOURS	**18**	**(15/6)**

Spring Semester		
PHSC 122 Medicinal Chemistry II	3	(3/0)
PHYS 121 Physiology	5	(4/1)
PHSC 123 Pharmaceutical Technology	5	(4/4)
MICR 211 Microbiology & Immunology	4	(3/2)
PPE 121 Basic Clinical & Communication Skills	2	(1/3)
TOTAL HOURS	**19**	**(15/10)**
FIRST YEAR TOTAL SEMESTER HOURS =	**37**	

SECOND PROFESSIONAL YEAR

Fall Semester	Semester Hours	Lecture/Laboratory
PHAR 211 Pharmacology I	4	(3/2)
PHSC 212 Parenterals	2	(1/3)
PHSC 221 Biopharmaceutics	3	(3/0)
PPE 211 Professional Practice Management	2	(2/0)
PPE 224 Introductory Clerkship	1	(0/2)
Elective(s)	4	(varies)
Total Hours	**16**	**(12/4)**

Spring Semester		
PHAR 221 Pharmacology II	4	(4/0)
PPE 221 Self-care & Nonprescription Drugs	3	(3/0)
CLPH 311 Therapeutics I	4	(4/0)
PPE 222 Drug Information & Literature Evaluation	2	(1/2)
PHSC 233 Pharmacokinetics	3	(2/2)
CLPH 324/325 Community/Institutional Rotation (May)	4	(0/10)
Elective(s)	2	(varies)
Total Hours	**22**	**(14/14)**

SECOND YEAR TOTAL SEMESTER HOURS = 38

THIRD PROFESSIONAL YEAR

Fall Semester	Semester Hours	Lecture/Laboratory
CLPH 312 Therapeutics II	4	(4/0)
CLPH 313 Therapeutics III	4	(4/0)
CLPH 314 Applied Therapeutics	2	(2/0)
CLPH 315 Applied Pharmacokinetics	3	(2/2)
PPE 213 Legal & Ethical Env. of Pharmacy	3	(3/0)
Elective(s)	2	(varies)
Total Hours	**18**	**(16/2)**

Spring Semester		
CLPH 321 Therapeutics IV	3	(3/0)
CLPH 322 Therapeutics V	3	(3/0)
PPE 223 Patient Assessment	2	(1/2)
CLPH 323 Applied Therapeutics II	2	(2/0)
PPE 324/325 Community/Institutional Rotation	4	(0/10)
Therapeutic Selective	2	(2/0)
Total Hours	**16**	**(11/12)**

THIRD YEAR TOTAL SEMESTER HOURS = 32

FOURTH PROFESSIONAL YEAR

Fall Semester	Semester Hours	Lecture/Laboratory
CLPH 411 Clinical Rotation I	4	(0/10)
CLPH 412 Clinical Rotation II	4	(0/10)
CLPH 413 Clinical Rotation III	4	(0/10)
CLPH 414 Clinical Rotation IV	4	(0/10)
CLPH 415 Clinical Rotation V	4	(0/10)
Total Hours	**20**	**(0/50)**

Spring Semester		
Rotation (selective)	4	(0/10)
Rotation (selective)	4	(0/10)
Rotation (selective)	4	(0/10)
Rotation (elective)	4	(0/10)
Rotation (elective)	4	(0/10)
Total Hours	**20**	**(0/50)**

FOURTH YEAR TOTAL SEMESTER HOURS = 40

As you will note from the above curricula, there is a significant amount of basic science course work, including biochemistry, anatomy, physiology, medical microbiology, as well as pharmaceutical chemistry and pharmacology. Other required courses may include nonprescription products, communication skills, toxicology, and drug literature evaluation.

The clinical science area of the curriculum deals with professional practice. The curriculum of the final professional year is heavily oriented toward pharmacy practice. Students participate in rotations (professional experience program), where they apply what they know (basic and pharmaceutical sciences) to actual pharmacy practice. At rotation sites, students are educated by practicing pharmacists alongside medical, nursing, and other health-care students in a "health-care team approach."

Students can obtain rotation experience in such settings as community pharmacies, drug information centers, adult medical units, pediatric units, psychiatric units, ambulatory clinics, long-term care facilities, pharmaceutical manufacturing firms, and nuclear pharmacies. At these sites, students provide a variety of services to patients, including dispensing medications, educating and monitoring patients about drug therapy, and conducting medication history interviews. Students may also serve as consultants, providing information to other health-care professionals about drug therapies.

Pharm.D. curricula require a minimum of 1,500 hours of professional practice experience. The University of Tennessee requires 1,960 hours of rotation experience. These hours are obtained by completing 12 one-month experiences of 160 hours per month. The amount of clinical experience required in a B.S. program is a minimum of 400 hours of rotation versus 1,500 hours in Pharm.D. programs.

For information on a pharmacy college's curriculum you should write to the dean's office of the college in which you are interested. The addresses of the colleges of pharmacy in the United States are listed in the Appendix.

FREQUENTLY ASKED QUESTIONS ABOUT PHARMACY EDUCATION

What are the job opportunities for a Doctor of Pharmacy graduate?

In addition to the jobs performed by B.S. graduates, the Pharm.D. graduate is qualified for highly specialized fields. (*Note:* At the annual meeting of the American Society of Hospital Pharmacists, December 2001, over 60 percent of the jobs posted in the placement service showed preference to Pharm.D. graduates over B.S. graduates.)

Can the Pharm.D. candidate specialize in a chosen area?

Most Pharm.D. programs offer students the opportunity for students to take electives and develop emphasis in areas such as pharmacokinetics, metabolic support, nuclear pharmacy, pediatrics, drug information, mental health, geriatrics, infectious disease, home health care, community pharmacy, industrial pharmacy, and other specialties.

Are post-doctoral residencies available?

There are a number of residency options available to graduates, including general hospital pharmacy residencies, specialty residencies, clinical residencies, and fellowships. A general residency or clinical residency is normally completed prior to the fellowship. Residencies are currently accredited by the American Society of Health-System Pharmacists (ASHP), and a number of new residency programs are being developed in community and other ambulatory-care settings. Residency descriptions and information can be obtained from the ASHP. Details about residency programs in the community are available from the American Pharmaceutical Association.

How will future roles of pharmacists differ from present roles?

The financing and organization of health care is changing rapidly. As the health-care system changes, so do the professions within the system. New laws in several states permit pharmacists to become actively involved in the prescribing of medications (collaborative-care agreements). There will be a continuous evolution of the pharmacist's role from dispenser of medications to health practitioner—with greater control over the selection and administration of medicines. Managed care and the market place are dictating major changes in the health-care system, and pharmacy is responding to those needs.

Do the anticipated changes in roles for the future necessitate a change in education?

Education will meet the future needs of the pharmacy practitioner. Greater emphasis is being placed on high technology, wellness care, self-care, computer applications, and other innovations in order to prepare pharmacists for new responsibilities. Doctor of Pharmacy degree programs have evolved over the years in response to changing demands for specialized instruction and training. More pharmacists are continuing in postgraduate education after their B.S. or Pharm.D. degrees to prepare themselves for specialty areas of practice.

What factors should be considered in selecting a program for a professional pharmacy education?

Choosing a college or school of pharmacy is an extremely important and often difficult decision. Many factors should be evaluated, but the primary goal is to select the program that offers the highest quality of education and level of service. The institution's commitment to academic excellence and concern for students' needs are important selection criteria. The location and setting are also key factors.

Chapter 2: Admission Process

REQUIREMENTS FOR ADMISSION

Each college/school of pharmacy has its own admissions requirements and deadlines. Contact the institution you are considering to determine the exact requirements.

Typically, each college/school requires a minimum of two years pre-pharmacy, three letters of reference, transcripts, a personnel interview, and a minimum score on the PCAT examination. Please note that some schools of pharmacy now require three years of pre-pharmacy, and at least one school requires a B.S. degree to be considered for admission.

The PCAT

If the college/school you are applying to requires the PCAT, you should take it in the Fall before you apply. This gives you the opportunity to retake the PCAT in the Winter if needed. Note that many colleges/schools of pharmacy do not penalize applicants for taking the test more than once and you can often use your highest score. Since PCAT requirements vary at each college/school, be sure to check with individual testing guidelines. You can usually take the PCAT until you receive a score that is above the minimum requirement of the institution to which you are applying. More information on the PCAT will be provided in Part II of this book.

HEALTH PROFESSION ADVISORS

Most colleges have health profession advisors who can assist in determining the courses that satisfy the requirements for admission to your school(s) of choice. If you are enrolled in an institution that does not have a college of pharmacy, you should seek advice from your health profession and pre-pharmacy advisors. For more information on health advisors, contact the National Association of Advisors for the Health Professions (NAAHP); P.O. Box 1518; Champaign, IL 61824-1518; phone: (217) 355-0063 or fax: (217) 355-1287.

APPLICATION PROCESS

The following steps should be considered when applying to a college of pharmacy:

1. Meet with or call the admissions officer to determine the requirements for admission.

2. Be sure that you meet the pre-pharmacy requirements of the college/school, or that you are on track to meet the requirements.

3. Make certain that your current transcripts are in order and that they are sent to the college by your registrar's office. *Note:* Be sure to update your transcript as you finish requirements since you will most likely have at least one semester of grades that are not on the submitted transcript.

4. Be sure that your pre-professional evaluations have been submitted to your home institution (this is done by your faculty advisor, pre-health advisor, or, in some institutions, by a professor in the student's major).

Letters of Recommendation

Letters from employers are preferred to determine your work ethic. Letters from professors are also desirable. If one professor is already involved in the pre-professional evaluation, other professors or employers should be used. For example, if you have worked for a pharmacist, or have a pharmacist who knows you well (i.e., is familiar with your academic status and work ethic), use this professional as a reference.

Do not submit letters from clergy or from political contacts unless the political contact is a relative or pharmacist.

Interviews

Many colleges/schools of pharmacy require interviews with students. These interviews are granted based on your PCAT scores and grade point average.

For your interview, you should:

1. Dress in business attire.

2. Be prepared to write a one-page essay (some schools require this, but not all).

3. Be honest and clear on why you want to enter the pharmacy profession.

4. Show that you are animated and excited about the profession.

5. Be prepared to discuss any issues in your academic background that would raise questions with the admissions committee.

FINANCIAL AID

There is a variety of financial aid available for students entering pharmacy programs. You may, for instance, be eligible for one or more of the following federal aid programs:

- Pell Grants (Federal funding available for students on a needs basis)

- College Work Study (Federal and local funds available to pay salaries for students working on campus)

- Supplemental Educational Opportunity Grants (SEOG)

- Health Professions Student Loans (HPSL)

- Health Education Assistance Loans (HEAL)

- Veterans' Benefits

- National Direct Student Loan Programs

- Federal Family Education Loans

For more information about eligibility for these programs and how you can apply, write to the U.S. Department of Education or call the Federal Student Aid Information Center at (800) 333-INFO.

In addition to federal programs, most colleges/schools of pharmacy offer need-based and/or merit scholarships to students. Each college or school also has its own financial aid program and may offer loans, grants, and scholarships. You should request financial aid information from each of the pharmacy programs to which you apply.

Many private foundations and organizations also have scholarship programs. Most libraries have directories listing foundations and other private grants to individuals. Libraries also carry reference volumes that describe in detail all forms and sources of financial aid for undergraduate, professional, and graduate study.

PHARMACY EDUCATION COSTS

Pharmacy education costs include tuition, fees, books, and housing—and vary by institution.

The following is an example of the costs for a pharmacy student entering the University of Tennessee College of Pharmacy in Memphis, Tennessee. These costs are based on estimates for the 2002–03 academic year.

University of Tennessee College of Pharmacy Resident

Expense	Estimated Cost
Resident Tuition and Fees	$9,000
Books and Supplies	750
Living Expenses	6,000
Total costs for one year	**$15,750**

Over four years, the total estimated costs without tuition or fee increases is $63,000.

University of Tennessee College of Pharmacy Non-Resident

Non-resident tuition and Fees	$19,000
Books and Supplies	750
Living Expenses	6,000
Travel	1,500
Total costs for one year	**$28,250**

Over four years, the total estimated costs without tuition or fee increases is $113,000.

Chapter 3: Postgraduate Education

RESIDENCIES

In 1953, the American Society of Health-System Pharmacists (ASHP) began the accreditation of postgraduate training programs in hospital pharmacy. These programs were called hospital pharmacy residencies. During the past twenty years, residency programs have proliferated. The ASHP is the accrediting body for hospital pharmacy residencies as well as specialty residencies. There are more than 183 accredited residency programs in the United States, as well as other non-accredited fellowship, residency, and specialty residency programs. This number is growing every year.

FREQUENTLY ASKED QUESTIONS ABOUT PHARMACY RESIDENCIES*

What is a pharmacy residency?

A pharmacy residency is an organized, directed postgraduate learning experience in a defined area of pharmacy practice.

What types of pharmacy residencies are there?

The most common type of residency is a pharmacy practice residency, conducted in an institution under the preceptorship of the director of the pharmacy department. The objective of residency training in pharmacy practice is to develop competent practitioners who are able to provide a broad scope of pharmaceutical services (clinical, informational, drug distribution, product formulation, quality control, supportive administrative, etc.). Training typically involves structured rotations within the pharmacy department and within other departments in the hospital, and includes participation in conferences, seminars, research projects, and related activities. Many residencies also provide limited experience in other hospital pharmacies or organized health-care settings.

Another type of residency is a specialty pharmacy practice area. It emphasizes the provision of pharmaceutical care to a wide variety of patients. Although most of the resident's training takes place in an institution, less emphasis is placed on the overall operation of a pharmacy department. Most specialty residencies are available only to those who have completed the Pharm.D. degree. These specialty residencies include psychiatry, drug information, pharmacokinetics, cardiology, geriatrics, pediatrics, nutrition, critical care, etc.

What is meant by an "accredited" residency?

The American Society of Health-Systems Pharmacists (ASHP) is the accrediting body for the types of residencies described above. The ASHP grants accreditation to institutions that meet certain standards of practice and demonstrate a quality-training program. Accreditation of a pharmacy residency program provides assurance to prospective residents that the program has met the basic requirements and is therefore an acceptable site for postgraduate training in pharmacy practice.

How many hours are required to complete a pharmacy residency?

A minimum of 2,000 hours of training extending over a minimum of fifty weeks is required in an ASHP-accredited residency program—the equivalent of one average work year. Some residency programs are offered only in conjunction with an advanced degree (M.S. or Pharm.D.) in a college of pharmacy or graduate school. Such programs are commonly referred to as "affiliated" residencies and generally require two years for completion. Residents in some affiliated programs pursue the residency on a part-time basis so there will be adequate time for course work, thesis research, and other degree requirements. Many affiliated programs, however, allow the residency to be taken either before or after the postgraduate academic course work.

Other residency programs ("nonaffiliated" residencies) are offered independently of an advanced degree and typically require one year of full-time work for completion. An applicant who already holds an advanced degree would normally choose one of these programs if he or she is interested in pursuing residency training.

Do residents earn a salary?

All accredited residency programs provide the resident with a stipend, although the amount varies from program to program, depending on the number of actual residency training hours per year, the value of any fringe benefits provided, and geographic location (cost of living). The stipends are generally inadequate to cover living costs for a resident having significant family support responsibilities. The average salary for residents in 2002-2003 was $34,000 per year. Furthermore, a residency, whether affiliated or nonaffiliated, requires a full-time commitment on the part of the resident and usually does not permit supplementing income through part-time employment. For these reasons, applicants with family support obligations should have financial resources in addition to the residency stipend upon which they can rely during the residency-training period.

Who should consider taking an accredited pharmacy residency?

Any pharmacist or pharmacy student whose career objectives center around institutional or clinical pharmacy practice should give serious consideration to residency training. Because of the concentrated nature of the training in a residency program, an individual may develop competence in a broader scope of pharmacy practice in a one- or two-year residency program than might be expected from several years as a staff pharmacist with a fixed assignment. Many "positions available" listings in the ASHP Personnel Placement Service specify completion of an accredited residency as an employment prerequisite.

What are the requirements for admission to an accredited pharmacy residency?

An applicant must be a graduate of an ACPE-accredited college of pharmacy (or must have graduated prior to the beginning date of the residency) and should have demonstrated an interest in and aptitude for advanced training in pharmacy. Some residencies require that the applicant be licensed to practice before entering the program, although others will accept applicants who have some limited internship obligation remaining for completion of state board licensure requirements. In the case of an affiliated residency program, the applicant must satisfy the requirements of the college of pharmacy or graduate school for admission to the advanced degree program, in addition to the requirements established by the institution in which the residency is offered. Residents in ASHP-accredited programs should be members of the American Society of Health-Systems Pharmacists. Students with B.S. or Pharm.D. degrees who are applying for postgraduate residency and/or fellowship programs should write to the American Society of Health-Systems Pharmacists Residency Matching Program, 7272 Wisconsin Avenue, Bethesda, MD 20814; phone: (301) 657-3000 or fax: (301) 652-8278; Web site: www.ashp.org. A list of accredited residencies may be obtained from the ASHP.

---

* *From the ASHP publication "What Is a Pharmacy Residency?" Reprinted with permission of the American Society of Health-Systems Pharmacists.*

FELLOWSHIPS

Fellowships focus on research in a specific area and usually require the completion of a residency. They are typically two years in length and are designed to prepare the fellow for a career in education or industry.

For more information contact:

The American College of Clinical Pharmacy
3101 Broadway, Suite 380
Kansas City, MO 64111
Phone: (816) 531-2177
Fax: (816) 531-4990
Web site: www.accp.com

GRADUATE EDUCATION

Graduate education in colleges of pharmacy can be broadly divided into two areas:

1. **Pharmaceutical Sciences:** This includes medicinal chemistry, pharmaceutics, pharmacokinetics, drug metabolism, pharmacology, and toxicology. M.S. and Ph.D. degrees are offered.

2. **Health Science Administration:** This area includes pharmacoeconomics, health policy, administration, practice management, and social and administrative science programs. M.S. and Ph.D. degrees are offered.

For more information contact:

The American Association of Colleges of Pharmacy
1426 Prince Street
Alexandria, VA 22314
Phone: (703) 739-2330
Fax: (703) 836-8982
Web site: www.aacp.org

PART II

Introduction to the PCAT

Chapter 4: Test Details

GENERAL INFORMATION ABOUT THE TEST

The Pharmacy College Admission Test (PCAT) is a national examination designed to measure the general ability and scientific knowledge of applicants seeking admission to selected schools and colleges of pharmacy. The PCAT is developed and administered by The Psychological Corporation under the auspices of the American Association of Colleges of Pharmacy. The test serves as a tool for admissions committees to compare information about the academic abilities of students.

You can obtain a booklet that describes the current fee structure and contains an application to take the PCAT for no charge from The Psychological Corporation. Direct your correspondence and requests for information about the PCAT to:

The Psychological Corporation
PSE Customer Relations—PCAT
19500 Bulverde Road
San Antonio, TX 78259
Phone: (800) 622-3231 or (210) 339-8710
Fax: (210) 339-8711 or (888) 211-8276
Monday–Friday, 8:30 a.m. to 5 p.m. Central Time

Be sure to include your name, address, Social Security number, and the name of the testing program when writing to The Psychological Corporation.

When the Test Is Given

The test is generally given three times a year in October, January or February, and April. Scores are available about four weeks after the test date. Contact The Psychological Corporation for exact dates as well as deadlines for submission of applications.

FEES AND SPECIAL SERVICES

The Psychological Corporation accepts fee payments by money order only. Make your money order payable to THE PYSCHOLOGICAL CORPORATION. If you are applying from outside the United States, you must submit an international money order payable in U.S. dollars.

Your application with all required fees must be received by the application deadline for the test date for which you are applying. Send your application and fee payments by regular mail to the following address:

The Psychological Corporation
Pharmacy College Admission Test
P.O. Box 91581
Chicago, IL 60693

If you need to use overnight courier service to meet the application and fee deadline, address it to:

The Psychological Corporation
c/o of Bank of America
91581 Collections Center Drive
Chicago, IL 60693

The following fee schedule is for the 2002–2003 academic year. For current rates please check with The Psychological Corporation.

Fee Schedule

Test Fee $69 (U.S.)

OPTIONAL FEES

Late Application Fee $31 (U.S.)

To apply after the regular deadline up to four weeks before the test, you must pay this fee in addition to the test fee.

Special Testing Location Fee $152 (U.S.)

To take your test at a location other than a scheduled testing center, you must pay this fee in addition to the test fee.

Standby Registration Fee $39 (U.S.)

If you do not preregister to take your test, you must pay this fee in addition to the test fee.

Additional Score Report Fee $16 (U.S.) Each

You must pay this fee for each score report beyond the three that your test fee covers, and for any requested score report after you submit your application.

Handscoring Fee $31 (U.S.)

To have your electronically-scored answer sheet rescored by hand to confirm your reported score, you must pay this additional fee.

TESTING LOCATIONS AND SPECIAL CONSIDERATIONS

Testing centers are located in every state of the United States and in locations throughout Canada. You should contact The Psychological Corporation for exact locations of testing centers.

Special testing locations for the established testing dates may be arranged for candidates living more than 150 miles from a scheduled testing center. For candidates whose religious convictions prohibit their testing on a Saturday, a special testing date on the Sunday following the scheduled test date may be arranged. The Psychological Corporation must receive requests for accommodations for candidates with disabilities by the application deadline that appears on the back cover of the Candidate Information Booklet provided by The Psychological Corporation.

TEST CONTENT

The PCAT is a multiple-choice test containing approximately 300 questions. Each question has four answer choices, only one of which is correct. The answer to any question can be derived independently of any other question. Students have approximately 3 hours and 30 minutes to complete the examination. This includes a short test break halfway through the test.

The PCAT is divided into five content areas with each area timed separately. During the time for a specific section, you are allowed to work on that section only. Once you have completed a section and have moved on to a new one, you are not allowed to go back to a previous section. While working on a section, it is advisable to answer those questions that are easy for you first, then go back and answer questions you find more difficult.

CONTENT AREAS

Verbal Ability—This area measures general, nonscientific word knowledge using antonyms and analogies.

Quantitative Ability—This area measures skills in arithmetic processes—including fractions, decimals, and percentages—and the ability to reason through and understand quantitative concepts and relationships, including applications of algebra. (Trigonometry and calculus are not included.)

Biology—This area measures knowledge of the principles and concepts of basic biology and human anatomy, with a major emphasis on human physiology.

Chemistry—This area measures knowledge of principles and concepts of inorganic and elementary organic chemistry. This includes application of formulas, interpretation of results, and chemistry problems.

Reading Comprehension—This area measures ability to comprehend, analyze, and interpret reading passages on scientific topics.

The order in which the sections are arranged on the actual PCAT test may not be the same as in this book. Note that the order of the sections change with different examinations and dates. The following chart indicates the approximate number of questions per section and the time allowed for each.

PCAT Content Area	App. Number of Questions	App. Time
Verbal Ability	50	30 minutes
Quantitative Ability	65	45 minutes
Biology	50	30 minutes
Chemistry	60	30 minutes
Reading Comprehension	45	45 minutes

PCAT SCORING

You will be sent your test scores approximately four weeks after taking the test. Scores are not faxed or reported over the telephone. The personal score report that you receive provides you with a total score, scaled score, and the percentile score. A composite score is then computed from the scaled score and percentile score.

The scaled score is calculated from the number of correct responses on each section of the PCAT. This means that you will not be penalized for incorrect answers. The scale ranges from approximately 100 to 300, with a median of 200 (i.e., a scaled score of 200 is equivalent to the 50th percentile). The Psychological Corporation does not set a passing or failing score for the PCAT examination. Acceptable scores are determined by each college/school.

The percentile score indicates the placement of your scaled score in the total pool of test-takers. The pool represents other students who took the test at the same time and factors in results from previous test administrations. It does not factor in your previous scaled score if you have taken the PCAT before. If you receive a 50 in the percentile column, this indicates that you did better than 50 percent of the other students in that content area, thus scoring in the 50th percentile. The percentile score reflects the percentage of applicants throughout the United States with lower scores on the respective section.

The composite score is an unweighted average of the five content area scores. Lower scores in the content areas pull the average down while higher scores in content areas pull the scores up. If you retake the PCAT, it is important to understand that you need to maintain the high scores you obtained in specific content areas while attempting to improve scores in other content areas. Be sure to contact the colleges/schools you are applying to find out how they interpret PCAT scores and how they evaluate repeat PCAT scores.

Chapter 5: Tips to Score High on the PCAT

STUDY PREPARATION

By answering the practice/review questions, you can determine your weakest areas and target what you need to review. Once you have completed your review, you should take the practice examination in this book under the following test-taking conditions:

- Time each section.

- Do not use study aids or refer to the answer key.

- Take the practice examination in a quiet place with no distractions.

- Concentrate on the practice examination as if it were the actual PCAT.

Here are eight general tips that will help you improve your PCAT scores. These tips can be used for PCAT or any other standardized national examination:

1. Get 8 hours of sleep the night before.

2. Know exactly where you have to go to take the examination.

3. Arrive at the testing site at least 30 minutes prior to the examination.

4. Utilize the practice/review materials in this book and take the practice examination under test conditions.

5. Be sure to bring at least 6 sharpened #2 pencils with erasers and a small hand pencil sharpener.

6. Bring an accurate watch or small clock (that does not make ticking noises).

7. Be sure to bring your picture identification with you to the testing site.

8. Be sure of your test date and that you have a confirmation for your test time and site.

TIME MANAGEMENT

Time management is very important on an examination such as the PCAT. The following is a list of things you can do to manage your time and improve your score on the PCAT:

1. Answer every question on the examination.

2. Familiarize yourself with the question types and directions for each content area.

3. Pace yourself and work within the allotted time given for each content area.

4. When you start a section, answer the questions that you know the answer to first.

5. Read over all of the answer choices before choosing your answer.

6. Remember that you can write on the examination book and make notes if you are unsure about a question or if you have not answered a question.

7. Do NOT make any stray marks on the examination answer sheet. If you do, make sure to erase them completely.

8. If you need to change an answer on your answer sheet, be sure to erase the answer completely.

9. Be sure to transfer each answer from the test book to the corresponding answer on the answer sheet. You should be careful to check your answer sheet against the test question to make sure they match.

10. Do NOT leave any answer blank. You are not penalized for guessing.

11. You cannot use a calculator on the PCAT. Practice the quantitative ability section without the use of a calculator.

12. Answer all of the practice/review questions and take the practice examination the day before you are scheduled for the PCAT.

PCAT SCORING RECAP

There are numerous reasons why students do not score well on standardized tests. These reasons include illness, stress, being late for the examination, and not having enough time to study and/or practice for the PCAT. Follow the tips in the previous section to help avoid these obstacles and improve your PCAT score.

As discussed in Chapter 4, the PCAT examination utilizes two scores on each section, a scaled score and a percentile score. The percentile and scaled scores are then reported as a composite score.

PCAT scores are computed based on the number of correct answers in each section. It is to your advantage to answer all questions even if you do not know an answer.

Percentile scores provide the admission committees at participating colleges and schools of pharmacy with a comparison of your scaled score to the total number of students taking the examination. Your previous test scores are not included in this score; therefore, you are not penalized for taking the examination more than once.

Composite scores include all five of the content areas and represent the average of the scaled scores from each of the content sections. It is important to remember that if you are taking the examination for the second or third time, you should study each content area, since your previous scores in an area are not included in the composite score. For example, if you score high on Quantitative Ability and low on Reading Comprehension the first time you take the PCAT, and then score low on Quantitative Ability and high on Reading Comprehension the second time you take the exam, you probably will not improve your overall score.

Most admissions committees recognize the composite percentile score as the best marker for comparison with other students. Check with the college or school to which you are applying to determine if they have a minimum score. Also, ask the admissions officer what the average score was for the entering class of the previous year. This will give you an idea of how you have to score to be successful in admission to the college/school of your choice.

WHEN TO TAKE THE PCAT

Find out the deadline for completed applications for the college/school(s) of pharmacy you are interested in. Allow yourself plenty of time to meet the deadlines. Do not wait until the last possible test date to take the PCAT.

Try to take the PCAT at least two to three test dates prior to the deadline for your completed admission portfolio in case you need to take the examination again prior to the school(s) admissions deadline. This is an important strategy to remember, since it will give you a chance to improve your score if needed.

How Many Times Should I Take the PCAT?

The number of times you should take the PCAT depends upon your score. If your score meets the criteria for the school(s) to which you are applying, and you are satisfied with the score, then you do not need to take the PCAT again. However, if your score does not meet the admissions criteria of the school(s) to which you have submitted applications, then you need to take the examination again.

Here are four factors involved in how many times you take the PCAT:

1. Your percentile score

2. If your score meets the admissions requirements of the school(s) where you have submitted applications

3. When you have taken enough pre-pharmacy courses to feel confident about taking the PCAT

4. If the school(s) to which you have submitted applications consider only the *highest* PCAT score, then take the PCAT until you are satisfied with your score

PART III

PCAT Review
and Practice Questions

Part III provides you with the review and practice you need to prepare for your PCAT test day. It includes *Key Points to Remember* about each content area and practice questions in each of the five PCAT content areas. Note that the number of practice questions does not reflect the actual number of test questions on the PCAT; there are more questions in this practice section than on the actual test. The number of practice questions is broken down as follows:

Content Area	Practice Questions
Verbal Ability	100
Quantitative Ability	100
Biology	75
Chemistry	100
Reading Comprehension	45

Chapters 6 through 10 are organized with *Key Points to Remember*, an *Answer Sheet*, *Practice Questions*, an *Answer Key*, and *Explanatory Answers* for each content area.

Chapter 6: Verbal Ability

Communication skills are important to the pharmacy profession, enabling pharmacists to provide comprehensive care to patients and to communicate effectively with other health-care providers. The ability to clearly express verbal and written thoughts is a desirable attribute for pharmacists. Many colleges/schools of pharmacy evaluate communication skills during the admissions interview. For example, the admissions committee may ask you to write a brief answer to a question or to write on a specific topic during the interview.

The Verbal Ability section evaluates and measures your vocabulary and your ability to analyze through the use of antonyms, synonyms, and analogy questions.

KEY POINTS TO REMEMBER

1. Synonyms are words that have the *same* or *nearly the same* meaning.

2. Antonyms are words that are *opposite* or *nearly the opposite* of each other in meaning.

3. Analogies are sets or pairs of words that describe a similar relationship; the relationship may be clear or may be somewhat obscure.

4. Analogy questions typically take longer to answer than synonym or antonym questions; therefore answer analogy questions last.

5. Look carefully at each word—identifying prefixes, suffixes, and parts of speech.

6. For *antonym* questions look for words that are the closest to being *opposite* in definition.

7. For *synonym* questions look for words that are the closest to being the *same* in definition.

8. There is only one right answer to a question.

9. If it helps, place the word (synonym or antonym) in a sentence or phrase. Does the sentence or phrase make sense?

10. Review each word carefully for spelling; remember a single letter can make the difference in definition.

11. Using the process of elimination, cross out the words that are either clearly not the opposite or clearly not the same.

12. Analogies refer to relationships. These relationships may be clear or maybe somewhat obscure.

13. Improve your vocabulary each day by spending a few minutes exercising your knowledge of words. One way to do this is by completing the daily crossword puzzle in your local newspaper.

Answer Sheet

Chapter 6: Verbal Ability

1. Ⓐ Ⓑ Ⓒ Ⓓ   21. Ⓐ Ⓑ Ⓒ Ⓓ   41. Ⓐ Ⓑ Ⓒ Ⓓ   61. Ⓐ Ⓑ Ⓒ Ⓓ   81. Ⓐ Ⓑ Ⓒ Ⓓ

2. Ⓐ Ⓑ Ⓒ Ⓓ   22. Ⓐ Ⓑ Ⓒ Ⓓ   42. Ⓐ Ⓑ Ⓒ Ⓓ   62. Ⓐ Ⓑ Ⓒ Ⓓ   82. Ⓐ Ⓑ Ⓒ Ⓓ

3. Ⓐ Ⓑ Ⓒ Ⓓ   23. Ⓐ Ⓑ Ⓒ Ⓓ   43. Ⓐ Ⓑ Ⓒ Ⓓ   63. Ⓐ Ⓑ Ⓒ Ⓓ   83. Ⓐ Ⓑ Ⓒ Ⓓ

4. Ⓐ Ⓑ Ⓒ Ⓓ   24. Ⓐ Ⓑ Ⓒ Ⓓ   44. Ⓐ Ⓑ Ⓒ Ⓓ   64. Ⓐ Ⓑ Ⓒ Ⓓ   84. Ⓐ Ⓑ Ⓒ Ⓓ

5. Ⓐ Ⓑ Ⓒ Ⓓ   25. Ⓐ Ⓑ Ⓒ Ⓓ   45. Ⓐ Ⓑ Ⓒ Ⓓ   65. Ⓐ Ⓑ Ⓒ Ⓓ   85. Ⓐ Ⓑ Ⓒ Ⓓ

6. Ⓐ Ⓑ Ⓒ Ⓓ   26. Ⓐ Ⓑ Ⓒ Ⓓ   46. Ⓐ Ⓑ Ⓒ Ⓓ   66. Ⓐ Ⓑ Ⓒ Ⓓ   86. Ⓐ Ⓑ Ⓒ Ⓓ

7. Ⓐ Ⓑ Ⓒ Ⓓ   27. Ⓐ Ⓑ Ⓒ Ⓓ   47. Ⓐ Ⓑ Ⓒ Ⓓ   67. Ⓐ Ⓑ Ⓒ Ⓓ   87. Ⓐ Ⓑ Ⓒ Ⓓ

8. Ⓐ Ⓑ Ⓒ Ⓓ   28. Ⓐ Ⓑ Ⓒ Ⓓ   48. Ⓐ Ⓑ Ⓒ Ⓓ   68. Ⓐ Ⓑ Ⓒ Ⓓ   88. Ⓐ Ⓑ Ⓒ Ⓓ

9. Ⓐ Ⓑ Ⓒ Ⓓ   29. Ⓐ Ⓑ Ⓒ Ⓓ   49. Ⓐ Ⓑ Ⓒ Ⓓ   69. Ⓐ Ⓑ Ⓒ Ⓓ   89. Ⓐ Ⓑ Ⓒ Ⓓ

10. Ⓐ Ⓑ Ⓒ Ⓓ   30. Ⓐ Ⓑ Ⓒ Ⓓ   50. Ⓐ Ⓑ Ⓒ Ⓓ   70. Ⓐ Ⓑ Ⓒ Ⓓ   90. Ⓐ Ⓑ Ⓒ Ⓓ

11. Ⓐ Ⓑ Ⓒ Ⓓ   31. Ⓐ Ⓑ Ⓒ Ⓓ   51. Ⓐ Ⓑ Ⓒ Ⓓ   71. Ⓐ Ⓑ Ⓒ Ⓓ   91. Ⓐ Ⓑ Ⓒ Ⓓ

12. Ⓐ Ⓑ Ⓒ Ⓓ   32. Ⓐ Ⓑ Ⓒ Ⓓ   52. Ⓐ Ⓑ Ⓒ Ⓓ   72. Ⓐ Ⓑ Ⓒ Ⓓ   92. Ⓐ Ⓑ Ⓒ Ⓓ

13. Ⓐ Ⓑ Ⓒ Ⓓ   33. Ⓐ Ⓑ Ⓒ Ⓓ   53. Ⓐ Ⓑ Ⓒ Ⓓ   73. Ⓐ Ⓑ Ⓒ Ⓓ   93. Ⓐ Ⓑ Ⓒ Ⓓ

14. Ⓐ Ⓑ Ⓒ Ⓓ   34. Ⓐ Ⓑ Ⓒ Ⓓ   54. Ⓐ Ⓑ Ⓒ Ⓓ   74. Ⓐ Ⓑ Ⓒ Ⓓ   94. Ⓐ Ⓑ Ⓒ Ⓓ

15. Ⓐ Ⓑ Ⓒ Ⓓ   35. Ⓐ Ⓑ Ⓒ Ⓓ   55. Ⓐ Ⓑ Ⓒ Ⓓ   75. Ⓐ Ⓑ Ⓒ Ⓓ   95. Ⓐ Ⓑ Ⓒ Ⓓ

16. Ⓐ Ⓑ Ⓒ Ⓓ   36. Ⓐ Ⓑ Ⓒ Ⓓ   56. Ⓐ Ⓑ Ⓒ Ⓓ   76. Ⓐ Ⓑ Ⓒ Ⓓ   96. Ⓐ Ⓑ Ⓒ Ⓓ

17. Ⓐ Ⓑ Ⓒ Ⓓ   37. Ⓐ Ⓑ Ⓒ Ⓓ   57. Ⓐ Ⓑ Ⓒ Ⓓ   77. Ⓐ Ⓑ Ⓒ Ⓓ   97. Ⓐ Ⓑ Ⓒ Ⓓ

18. Ⓐ Ⓑ Ⓒ Ⓓ   38. Ⓐ Ⓑ Ⓒ Ⓓ   58. Ⓐ Ⓑ Ⓒ Ⓓ   78. Ⓐ Ⓑ Ⓒ Ⓓ   98. Ⓐ Ⓑ Ⓒ Ⓓ

19. Ⓐ Ⓑ Ⓒ Ⓓ   39. Ⓐ Ⓑ Ⓒ Ⓓ   59. Ⓐ Ⓑ Ⓒ Ⓓ   79. Ⓐ Ⓑ Ⓒ Ⓓ   99. Ⓐ Ⓑ Ⓒ Ⓓ

20. Ⓐ Ⓑ Ⓒ Ⓓ   40. Ⓐ Ⓑ Ⓒ Ⓓ   60. Ⓐ Ⓑ Ⓒ Ⓓ   80. Ⓐ Ⓑ Ⓒ Ⓓ   100. Ⓐ Ⓑ Ⓒ Ⓓ

Tear Here

Verbal Ability Practice Questions

100 QUESTIONS—1 HOUR

Directions: For questions 1–50, choose the lettered word that best completes the analogy.

1. CARDINAL : PRIMARY :: SECONDARY :
   - (A) tertiary
   - (B) subordinate
   - (C) pivotal
   - (D) key

2. AWAKE : ALIVE :: ASLEEP :
   - (A) arouse
   - (B) defunct
   - (C) functional
   - (D) excited

3. TACT : SAVOIR FAIRE :: COARSE :
   - (A) act
   - (B) diplomacy
   - (C) crude
   - (D) expert

4. EXPERT : ADEPT :: AMATEUR :
   - (A) dabbler
   - (B) beginner
   - (C) authority
   - (D) crackerjack

5. ACCOUNT : DEEM :: UNDERVALUE :
   - (A) consider
   - (B) re-guard
   - (C) view
   - (D) depreciate

6. SEQUELA : RESULT :: PRIMARY :
   - (A) secondary
   - (B) end
   - (C) aftereffect
   - (D) basis

7. BULLETIN : BOARD :: ANNOUNCEMENT :
   - (A) mail
   - (B) telephone
   - (C) newt
   - (D) bullet

8. BRIDLE : RESTRAIN :: JAIL :
   - (A) bridge
   - (B) marry
   - (C) lockup
   - (D) center

9. CONTAMINATE : POLLUTE :: WRECK :
   - (A) crash
   - (B) contemplate
   - (C) contain
   - (D) purify

10. DISPLEASURE : PIQUE :: PLEASURE :
    - (A) joy
    - (B) disposal
    - (C) madness
    - (D) bitterness

11. EVENTUATE : ENSUE :: UNDOUBTED :
    (A) end
    (B) entwine
    (C) crease
    (D) authentic

12. MAGNIFICENCE : GRANDIOSITY :: SCHNOOK :
    (A) fame
    (B) magnifier
    (C) dunce
    (D) magnitude

13. UNDULATE : STILL :: RETREAT :
    (A) poll
    (B) charge
    (C) free
    (D) retch

14. PARSIMONIOUS : SCROOGE :: LINCOLN :
    (A) miserly
    (B) liberal
    (C) conservative
    (D) genuine

15. QUIESCENT : DORMANT :: MOBILE :
    (A) auto
    (B) running
    (C) plane
    (D) quick

16. RADIOACTIVITY : RADIATION :: RADIO :
    (A) frequency
    (B) place
    (C) radar
    (D) ion

17. DEAN : STUDENT :: WIFE :
    (A) group
    (B) associate
    (C) son
    (D) relative

18. FLANK : END :: FEET :
    (A) side
    (B) meter
    (C) head
    (D) inches

19. DIPSOMANIAC : ALCOHOL :: ADDICT :
    (A) diplomat
    (B) insomniac
    (C) addiction
    (D) morphine

20. CORSAGE : NOSEGAY :: BUTLER :
    (A) maid
    (B) valet
    (C) receptionist
    (D) corset

21. CORTEGE : RETINUE :: LANE :
    (A) roadway
    (B) median
    (C) line
    (D) lineation

22. JOWL : JAW :: PIG :
    (A) head
    (B) cow
    (C) porcine
    (D) mule

23. SURMOUNT : CONQUER :: VICTORY :
   (A) survey
   (B) conquest
   (C) suspect
   (D) recount

24. PLIABLE : FLEXIBLE :: AGILE :
   (A) supple
   (B) scrupulous
   (C) programmable
   (D) reliable

25. ZEAL : INDIFFERENCE :: FERVOR :
   (A) foolishness
   (B) bright
   (C) pleasure
   (D) mute

26. TRANSCEND : LAG :: DUNCE :
   (A) overtake
   (B) pass
   (C) exceed
   (D) brainy

27. SHREWD : CALCULATING :: ODD :
   (A) cagey
   (B) strange
   (C) shrinkable
   (D) even

28. EXPENDITURE : DISBURSEMENT :: OVOLO :
   (A) credit
   (B) molding
   (C) debit
   (D) roe

29. EXPEDIENCY : RESOURCE :: EXPECT :
   (A) excellence
   (B) expulsion
   (C) efficiency
   (D) count

30. BEGUILE : DECEIVE :: DEPART :
   (A) become
   (B) envy
   (C) withdraw
   (D) enrage

31. *EXODUS* : BOOK :: BATMAN :
   (A) comics
   (B) radio
   (C) television
   (D) report

32. DENOUNCE : EULOGIZE :: PRODIGALITY :
   (A) parsimonious
   (B) impeach
   (C) connote
   (D) express

33. DENUDE : PEEL :: PROGRESS :
   (A) headway
   (B) cancel
   (C) depart
   (D) depress

34. CIRCUMSCRIBE : LIMIT :: PROGRAMMA :
   (A) chasten
   (B) circulate
   (C) agenda
   (D) launch

35. DEVIANT : NORMAL :: STARVE :
- **(A)** aberrant
- **(B)** suckle
- **(C)** nontitled
- **(D)** ghostly

36. MELEE : SKIRMISH :: INNING :
- **(A)** agreement
- **(B)** melange
- **(C)** frame
- **(D)** merger

37. ENIGMA : MYSTERY :: NOVEL :
- **(A)** enemy
- **(B)** neoteric
- **(C)** mark
- **(D)** imprecation

38. PALPABLE : TOUCHABLE :: SOFT :
- **(A)** pulpy
- **(B)** pristine
- **(C)** hard
- **(D)** tactful

39. RUDIMENTARY : ELEMENTAL :: RUDE :
- **(A)** parcel
- **(B)** civil
- **(C)** urbane
- **(D)** crude

40. IMPUGN : DESTROY :: LOVED :
- **(A)** deny
- **(B)** adored
- **(C)** implant
- **(D)** return

41. VALIDATE : ABROGATE : CONFIRM :
- **(A)** contradict
- **(B)** accede
- **(C)** assent
- **(D)** validate

42. TARIFF : DUTY :: TAUNT :
- **(A)** post
- **(B)** slack
- **(C)** goal
- **(D)** deride

43. WASTREL : VANGUARD :: MISER :
- **(A)** vagrant
- **(B)** spendthrift
- **(C)** wrangler
- **(D)** straggler

44. YAHOO : RUFFIAN :: MILKSOP :
- **(A)** yak
- **(B)** doormat
- **(C)** macho
- **(D)** gravy

45. SUAVE : URBANE :: RAMPART :
- **(A)** blues
- **(B)** foolish
- **(C)** bastion
- **(D)** urban

46. REMORSELESS : IMPENITENT :: IMPEND :
- **(A)** loom
- **(B)** remorseful
- **(C)** impatient
- **(D)** regretful

47. PERSNICKETY : FASTIDIOUS ::
    PERSUADABLE :
    (A) easy
    (B) pernicious
    (C) chancy
    (D) receptive

48. PERIMETER : INNERMORE :: EXTERNAL :
    (A) period
    (B) internal
    (C) area
    (D) end zone

49. IMPERIOUS : GENTLE :: GROVELING :
    (A) kindly
    (B) domineering
    (C) considerate
    (D) domestic

50. COMPASSION : SYMPATHY :: DOODLE :
    (A) unconcern
    (B) implacability
    (C) relentlessness
    (D) imbecile

Directions: For questions 51–100, choose the lettered word that means the *opposite* or *most nearly the opposite* of the word in capital letters.

51. DIFFICULTY
    (A) hardship
    (B) burden
    (C) trouble
    (D) effortlessness

52. IDEALISM
    (A) utopianism
    (B) realism
    (C) romanticism
    (D) perfectionism

53. HYSTERICAL
    (A) overwrought
    (B) calm
    (C) worked up
    (D) crazy

54. WELCOME
    (A) hello
    (B) good-bye
    (C) greeting
    (D) salutation

55. AFFLUENT
    (A) glamorous
    (B) stable
    (C) charitable
    (D) scanty

56. EXTRANEOUS
    (A) alien
    (B) foreign
    (C) extrinsic
    (D) intrinsic

57. VULNERABLE
    (A) reverent
    (B) innocent
    (C) unassailable
    (D) inflated

58. TAME
- **(A)** docile
- **(B)** submissive
- **(C)** calm
- **(D)** fierce

59. MAELSTROM
- **(A)** whirl
- **(B)** tranquility
- **(C)** fury
- **(D)** storm

60. NEFARIOUS
- **(A)** corrupt
- **(B)** degenerate
- **(C)** respectable
- **(D)** putrid

61. OPPORTUNE
- **(A)** suitable
- **(B)** tardy
- **(C)** seasonable
- **(D)** timely

62. DIVERSE
- **(A)** similar
- **(B)** definite
- **(C)** happy
- **(D)** cooperative

63. QUASH
- **(A)** abrogate
- **(B)** dissolve
- **(C)** initiate
- **(D)** quell

64. CAUSTIC
- **(A)** sleepy
- **(B)** sharp
- **(C)** unintelligent
- **(D)** soothing

65. ANIMATION
- **(A)** rebirth
- **(B)** evisceration
- **(C)** evaluation
- **(D)** revivification

66. REMONSTRATION
- **(A)** challenge
- **(B)** acquiescence
- **(C)** difficulty
- **(D)** demurral

67. ECLECTIC
- **(A)** selective
- **(B)** discriminating
- **(C)** picky
- **(D)** homogenous

68. FAMOUS
- **(A)** undistinguished
- **(B)** celebrated
- **(C)** redoubtable
- **(D)** prestigious

69. GLUTTONOUS
- **(A)** famished
- **(B)** rapacious
- **(C)** abstemious
- **(D)** ravenous

70. GLOAMING

    (A) evening

    (B) morning

    (C) twilight

    (D) eventide

71. TREPIDATION

    (A) honesty

    (B) fearlessness

    (C) anger

    (D) vigor

72. GLIMPSE

    (A) gander

    (B) glance

    (C) peek

    (D) peer

73. GLOOMY

    (A) bright

    (B) unhappy

    (C) dark

    (D) murky

74. INDOLENT

    (A) opulent

    (B) corpulent

    (C) lazy

    (D) industrious

75. JOVIALITY

    (A) mirth

    (B) hilarity

    (C) melancholy

    (D) jollity

76. SAGE

    (A) savant

    (B) buffoon

    (C) scholar

    (D) wise man

77. LISSOME

    (A) rigid

    (B) supple

    (C) lithe

    (D) limber

78. OBDURATE

    (A) callous

    (B) coldhearted

    (C) tender

    (D) mulish

79. OBSTREPEROUS

    (A) blatant

    (B) timorous

    (C) clamorous

    (D) vociferous

80. VALEDICTION

    (A) epistle

    (B) generosity

    (C) greeting

    (D) insecurity

81. OPEN-AIR

    (A) outside

    (B) inside

    (C) alfresco

    (D) outdoor

82. ODIOUS
    (A) hateful
    (B) sinful
    (C) spiteful
    (D) inoffensive

83. BUOYANCY
    (A) ebullience
    (B) effervescence
    (C) despondence
    (D) exuberance

84. RESCIND
    (A) reinstate
    (B) cancel
    (C) mutilate
    (D) recall

85. ENTHRALLED
    (A) flimsy
    (B) empty
    (C) bored
    (D) weak

86. SENILE
    (A) keen
    (B) ancient
    (C) senescent
    (D) decrepit

87. CHASTISE
    (A) cleanse
    (B) praise
    (C) straighten
    (D) reprove

88. TEMERITY
    (A) daring
    (B) caution
    (C) adventurousness
    (D) audacity

89. MULTICOLORED
    (A) variegated
    (B) parti-colored
    (C) versicolored
    (D) monochromatic

90. MODIFY
    (A) change
    (B) alter
    (C) vary
    (D) continue

91. FUROR
    (A) frenzy
    (B) serenity
    (C) stir
    (D) whirl

92. CONCILIATE
    (A) antagonize
    (B) pacify
    (C) appease
    (D) reconcile

93. DESCENDANT
    (A) kin
    (B) ancestor
    (C) seed
    (D) progeny

94. FAIR

   (A) just

   (B) equitable

   (C) unbiased

   (D) biased

95. LASCIVIOUS

   (A) lewd

   (B) libertine

   (C) puritan

   (D) salacious

96. ACCESSIBLE

   (A) remarkable

   (B) salable

   (C) unavailable

   (D) obtainable

97. REBUKE

   (A) reclaim

   (B) commend

   (C) reproach

   (D) complain

98. MOTLEY

   (A) hodgepodge

   (B) uniform

   (C) jumbled

   (D) mixed

99. IMPROMPTU

   (A) unplanned

   (B) extemporaneous

   (C) improvisational

   (D) rehearsed

100. WHIMSICAL

   (A) vagarious

   (B) whimsied

   (C) steadfast

   (D) capricious

ANSWER KEY

Verbal Ability									
1.	B	21.	A	41.	A	61.	B	81.	B
2.	B	22.	C	42.	D	62.	A	82.	D
3.	C	23.	B	43.	B	63.	C	83.	C
4.	A	24.	A	44.	B	64.	D	84.	A
5.	D	25.	D	45.	C	65.	B	85.	C
6.	D	26.	D	46.	A	66.	B	86.	A
7.	A	27.	B	47.	D	67.	D	87.	B
8.	C	28.	B	48.	B	68.	A	88.	B
9.	A	29.	D	49.	B	69.	C	89.	D
10.	A	30.	C	50.	D	70.	B	90.	D
11.	D	31.	A	51.	D	71.	B	91.	B
12.	C	32.	A	52.	B	72.	D	92.	A
13.	B	33.	A	53.	B	73.	A	93.	B
14.	D	34.	C	54.	B	74.	D	94.	D
15.	B	35.	B	55.	D	75.	C	95.	C
16.	A	36.	C	56.	D	76.	B	96.	C
17.	C	37.	B	57.	C	77.	A	97.	B
18.	C	38.	A	58.	D	78.	C	98.	B
19.	D	39.	D	59.	B	79.	B	99.	D
20.	B	40.	B	60.	C	80.	C	100.	C

EXPLANATORY ANSWERS

The Verbal Ability section answers include the corresponding correct answer (the word that best completes the analogy for questions 1–50 and the word that is opposite in meaning for questions 51–100), as well as the part of speech: noun (n.), verb (v.), adverb (adv.), or adjective (adj.).

1. **The correct answer is (B).**

    SECONDARY (n.)—one occupying a subordinate or auxiliary position rather than that of a principal. *Subordinate* (n.)—one that is placed in or occupying a lower class, rank, or position.

2. **The correct answer is (B).**

    ASLEEP (adj., adv.)—into a state of inactivity, sluggishness, or indifference. *Defunct* (adj.)—no longer living, existing, or functioning.

3. **The correct answer is (C).**

    COARSE (adj.)—of ordinary or inferior quality or value. *Crude* (adj.)—rough or inexpert in plan or execution.

4. **The correct answer is (A).**

    AMATEUR (n.)—one who engages in a pursuit, study, science, or sport as a pastime rather than as a profession. *Dabbler* (n.)—one that dabbles—as (adj.): one not deeply engaged in or concerned with something.

5. **The correct answer is (D).**

    UNDERVALUE (v.)—to value, rate, or estimate below the real worth. *Depreciate* (v.)—to lower in estimation or esteem.

6. **The correct answer is (D).**

    PRIMARY (n.)—something that stands first in rank, importance, or value. *Basis* (n.)—a supporting element; foundation.

7. **The correct answer is (A).**

    ANNOUNCEMENT (n.)—a public notification or declaration; a piece of formal stationery designed for a social or business announcement. *Mail* (n.)—materials, such as letters and packages, handled in a postal system.

8. **The correct answer is (C).**

    JAIL (n.)—a place of confinement for people held in lawful custody. *Lockup* (n.)—a jail.

9. **The correct answer is (A).**

    WRECK (n.)—the broken remains of something wrecked or otherwise ruined. *Crash* (n.)—to fall or collide noisily; smash.

10. **The correct answer is (A).**

    PLEASURE (n.)—a source of delight or joy. *Joy* (n.)—a condition or feeling of great pleasure.

11. **The correct answer is (D).**

UNDOUBTED (adj.)—not doubted; genuine; undisputed. *Authentic* (adj.)—conforming to fact and therefore worthy of trust.

12. **The correct answer is (C).**

SCHNOOK (n.)—a stupid or unimportant person. *Dunce* (n.)—one who is slow-witted or stupid.

13. **The correct answer is (B).**

RETREAT (n.)—an act or process of withdrawing especially from what is difficult, dangerous, or disagreeable. *Charge* (v., n.)—to rush forward in or as in a violent attack.

14. **The correct answer is (D).**

LINCOLN (n.)—Abraham Lincoln 1809-1865, sixteenth president of the United States (1861-65), known for his honesty and loyalty. *Genuine* (adj.)—free from hypocrisy or dishonesty.

15. **The correct answer is (B).**

MOBILE (adj.)—capable of moving or being moved. *Running* (n., v.)—the act or action of one that runs.

16. **The correct answer is (A).**

RADIO (n.)—the wireless transmission and reception of electric impulses or signals by means of electromagnetic waves. *Frequency* (n.)—the number of repetitions per unit time of a complete waveform.

17. **The correct answer is (C).**

WIFE (n.)—a female partner in a marriage. *Son* (n.)—a male offspring.

18. **The correct answer is (C).**

FEET (n.)—the terminal part of the vertebrate leg upon which an individual stands. *Head* (n., adj., v.)—the upper most or forward most part of the body.

19. **The correct answer is (D).**

ADDICT (v.)—to devote or surrender (oneself) to something habitually or obsessively. *Morphine* (n.)—an organic compound that is addictive; used for pain relief.

20. **The correct answer is (B).**

BUTLER (n.)—the chief male servant of a household, who has charge of other employees, receives guests, directs the serving of meals, and performs various personal services. *Valet* (n.)—to act as a personal servant.

21. **The correct answer is (A).**

LANE (n.)—a relatively narrow way or track. *Roadway* (n.)—the strip of land over which a road passes.

22. **The correct answer is (C).**

PIG (n.)—a young swine not yet sexually mature. *Porcine* (adj.)—relating to or suggesting swine.

23. **The correct answer is (B).**

   VICTORY (n.)—the overcoming of an enemy or antagonist. *Conquest* (n.)—the act or process of conquering.

24. **The correct answer is (A).**

   AGILE (adj.)—marked by ready ability to move with quick easy grace. *Supple* (adj.)—to make flexible or pliant.

25. **The correct answer is (D).**

   FERVOR (n.)—intensity of feeling or expression. *Mute* (n., adj.)—to tone down.

26. **The correct answer is (D).**

   DUNCE (n.)—a person dull or weak in intellect. *Brainy* (adj.)—having a well-developed intellect.

27. **The correct answer is (B).**

   ODD (adj.)—deviating from what is ordinary, usual, or expected. *Strange* (adj.)—not native to or naturally belonging to a place.

28. **The correct answer is (B).**

   OVOLO (n.)—a rounded convex molding. *Molding* (n.)—a decorative plane or curved strip used for ornamentation or finishing.

29. **The correct answer is (D).**

   EXPECT (v.)—to regard something as probable or likely. COUNT (v.)—to rely or depend on someone or something.

30. **The correct answer is (C).**

   DEPART (v.)—to go away; leave. *Withdraw* (v.)—to remove oneself from participation.

31. **The correct answer is (A).**

   BATMAN (n.)—comic book character name. *Comics* (n.)—the parts of a newspaper devoted to comic strips, a book of comic strips.

32. **The correct answer is (A).**

   PRODIGALITY (n.)—profuse generosity. *Parsimonious* (adj.)—frugal to the point of stinginess.

33. **The correct answer is (A).**

   PROGRESS (v.)—to advance or proceed. *Headway* (n.)—motion or rate of motion in a forward direction.

34. **The correct answer is (C).**

   PROGRAMMA (n.)—an edict published for public information. *Agenda* (n.)—a list, outline, or plan of things to be considered or done.

35. **The correct answer is (B).**

    STARVE (v.)—to suffer or die from extreme or prolonged lack of food. *Suckle* (v.)—to give milk to from the breast.

36. **The correct answer is (C).**

    INNING (n.)—a period of play in baseball during which each team has a turn at bat. *Frame* (n., v.)—something composed of parts fitted together and united.

37. **The correct answer is (B).**

    NOVEL (adj.)—strikingly new, unusual, or different. *Neoteric* (adj.)—recent in origin.

38. **The correct answer is (A).**

    SOFT (adj.)—smooth or fine to the touch. *Pulpy* (adj.)—the soft part of fruit.

39. **The correct answer is (D).**

    RUDE (adj.)—being in a crude, rough, unfinished condition. *Crude* (adj.)—marked by the primitive, gross, or elemental.

40. **The correct answer is (B).**

    LOVED (v.)—to have a deep feeling of affection and solicitude toward. *Adored* (v.)—to be extremely fond of.

41. **The correct answer is (A).**

    CONFIRM (v.)—to support or establish the certainty or validity of. *Contradict* (v.)—to resist or oppose in argument.

42. **The correct answer is (D).**

    TAUNT (v.)—to reproach in a mocking, insulting, or contemptuous manner. *Deride* (v.)—to laugh at contemptuously.

43. **The correct answer is (B).**

    MISER (n.)—one who lives very meagerly in order to hoard money. *Spendthrift* (n.)—one that spends improvidently or wastefully.

44. **The correct answer is (B).**

    MILKSOP (n.)—a timid man or boy considered childish or unassertive. *Doormat* (n.)—one that submits without protest to abuse or indignities.

45. **The correct answer is (C).**

    RAMPART (n.)—a fortification consisting of an embankment. *Bastion* (n.)—a projecting part of a fortification.

46. **The correct answer is (A).**

    IMPEND (v.)—to be imminent or about to happen. *Loom* (v.)—to take shape as an impending occurrence.

47. **The correct answer is (D).**

    PERSUADABLE (adj.)—being susceptible to persuasion. *Receptive* (adj.)—able or inclined to receive.

48. The correct answer is (B).

EXTERNAL (adj.)—relating to, existing on, or connected with the outside or an outer part; exterior. *Internal* (adj.)—existing or situated within the limits or surface of something.

49. The correct answer is (B).

GROVELING (adj.)—totally submissive. *Domineering* (adj.)—inclined to domineer.

50. The correct answer is (D).

DOODLE (n.)—a trifler; a simple fellow. *Imbecile* (n.)—a mentally deficient person.

51. The correct answer is (D).

DIFFICULTY (n.)—the quality or state of being difficult; something difficult. *Effortlessness* (n.)—showing or requiring little or no effort.

52. The correct answer is (B).

IDEALISM (n.)—the theory that true reality is in a realm beyond the form and all the phenomena; the practice of forming ideals or living under their influence. *Realism* (n.)—concern for fact or reality and rejection of the impractical and visionary.

53. The correct answer is (B).

HYSTERICAL (adj.)—characterized by unmanageable fear or emotional excess. *Calm* (adj.)—still; free from agitation, excitement, or disturbance.

54. The correct answer is (B).

WELCOME (n.)—a greeting or cordial remark made upon the entrance or arrival of a guest. *Good-bye* (n.)—an ending remark made to one who is leaving.

55. The correct answer is (D).

AFFLUENT (adj.)—flowing freely; plentiful or abundant. *Scanty* (adj.)—meager or insufficient.

56. The correct answer is (D).

EXTRANEOUS (adj.)—existing on the outside; not forming an essential part. *Intrinsic* (adj.)—belonging to the real nature of something; inherent.

57. The correct answer is (C).

VULNERABLE (adj.)—open to attack or easily hurt. *Unassailable* (adj.)—cannot be successfully attacked.

58. The correct answer is (D).

TAME (adj.)—calm or changed from a state of being wild to a domestic state. *Fierce* (adj.)—hostile in disposition; given to fighting.

59. The correct answer is (B).

MAELSTROM (n.)—a violently confused or agitated state of affairs. *Tranquility* (n.)—serenity or calmness.

60. **The correct answer is (C).**

   NEFARIOUS (adj.)—flagrantly wicked or impious. *Respectable* (adj.)—worthy of esteem.

61. **The correct answer is (B).**

   OPPORTUNE (adj.)—happening at the right time. *Tardy* (adj.)—behind time or late.

62. **The correct answer is (A).**

   DIVERSE (adj.)—different or varied. *Similar* (adj.)—nearly the same.

63. **The correct answer is (C).**

   QUASH (v.)—to nullify, suppress summarily and completely. *Initiate* (v.)—to bring into practice or use; to introduce.

64. **The correct answer is (D).**

   CAUSTIC (adj.)—corrosive; sarcastic or biting. *Soothing* (adj.)—calming; allaying or relieving pain.

65. **The correct answer is (B).**

   ANIMATION (n.)—the act of giving life or spirit to. *Evisceration* (n.)—the taking away of vital force.

66. **The correct answer is (B).**

   REMONSTRATION (n.)—protestation; presentation of reasons for opposition. *Acquiescence* (n.)—the act of accepting without objection.

67. **The correct answer is (D).**

   ECLECTIC (adj.)—composed of elements drawn from various sources. *Homogeneous* (adj.)—of uniform structure throughout.

68. **The correct answer is (A).**

   FAMOUS (adj.)—honored for outstanding achievement; widely known. *Undistinguished* (adj.)—not marked by any distinction.

69. **The correct answer is (C).**

   GLUTTONOUS (adj.)—excessive in eating or drinking. *Abstemious* (adj.)—sparing, especially in eating or drinking.

70. **The correct answer is (B).**

   GLOAMING (n.)—twilight. *Morning* (n.)—dawn; the time from sunrise to noon.

71. **The correct answer is (B).**

   TREPIDATION (n.)—fearful uncertainty; anxiety. *Fearlessness* (n.)—bravery or lack of fear.

72. **The correct answer is (D).**

   GLIMPSE (v.)—to take a brief look. *Peer* (v.)—to look searchingly at something.

73. **The correct answer is (A).**

   GLOOMY (adj.)—partially or totally dark; dismally dark. *Bright* (adj.)—full of light.

74. The correct answer is (D).

INDOLENT (adj.)—disliking or avoiding work. *Industrious* (adj.)—hardworking or diligent.

75. The correct answer is (C).

JOVIALITY (n.)—state of being markedly good humored, convivial, merry. *Melancholy* (n.)—depression.

76. The correct answer is (B).

SAGE (n.)—one distinguished for wisdom and sound judgment. *Buffoon* (n.)—one who is always clowning.

77. The correct answer is (A).

LISSOME (adj.)—lithe or nimble. *Rigid* (adj.)—not flexible; stiff and unyielding.

78. The correct answer is (C).

OBDURATE (adj.)—hardened in feelings; resistant to persuasion or softening influences. *Tender* (adj.)—having a soft or yielding nature.

79. The correct answer is (B).

OBSTREPEROUS (adj.)—unruly; marked by unruliness or aggressiveness. *Timorous* (adj.)—fearful or timid.

80. The correct answer is (C).

VALEDICTION (n.)—a good-bye; the act of saying farewell. *Greeting* (n.)—a reception or welcome.

81. The correct answer is (B).

OPEN-AIR (adj.)—outdoor. *Inside* (adj.)—of, relating to, or being on or near the inside.

82. The correct answer is (D).

ODIOUS (adj.)—disgusting, offensive, hateful. *Inoffensive* (adj.)—causing no harm or annoyance.

83. The correct answer is (C).

BUOYANCE (n.)—the tendency of a body to float or rise when submerged in a fluid; lightness or resilience of spirit; cheerfulness. *Despondence* (n.)—dejection or loss of hope.

84. The correct answer is (A).

RESCIND (v.)—to revoke or cancel. *Reinstate* (v.)—to restore to a former condition.

85. The correct answer is (C).

ENTHRALLED (adj.)—to be held spellbound or to be captivated by something. *Bored* (adj.)—to find dull and uninteresting.

86. The correct answer is (A).

SENILE (adj.)—exhibiting a loss of mental faculties associated with old age. *Keen* (adj.)—showing quick and ardent responsiveness.

87. The correct answer is (B).
CHASTISE (v.)—to punish; to scold or condemn sharply. *Praise* (v.)—to commend.

88. The correct answer is (B).
TEMERITY (n.)—unreasonable or fool-hardy contempt of danger or opposition; rashness; reckless-ness. *Caution* (n.)—wariness; prudent forethought to minimize risk.

89. The correct answer is (D).
MULTICOLORED (adj.)—displaying a variety of colors. *Monochromatic* (adj.)—of one color.

90. The correct answer is (D).
MODIFY (v.)—to make changes in. *Continue* (v.)—to keep the same; to maintain without interrup-tion.

91. The correct answer is (B).
FUROR (n.)—fury or rage. *Serenity* (n.)—calmness or tranquility.

92. The correct answer is (A).
CONCILIATE (v.)—to make compatible; to reconcile. *Antagonize* (v.)—to incur or provoke the hostility of.

93. The correct answer is (B).
DESCENDANT (n.)—one descended from another. *Ancestor* (n.)—a person from whom one is descended.

94. The correct answer is (D).
FAIR (n.)—free from bias; equitable. *Biased* (adj.)—prejudiced.

95. The correct answer is (C).
LASCIVIOUS (adj.)—lewd, lustful. *Puritan* (adj.)—relating to the Puritans or Puritanism; morally strict.

96. The correct answer is (C).
ACCESSIBLE (adj.)—obtainable. *Unavailable* (adj.)—not available.

97. The correct answer is (B).
REBUKE (v.)—to scold or reprimand. *Commend* (v.)—to express approval of or to praise.

98. The correct answer is (B).
MOTLEY (adj.)—composed of many colors or many different elements. *Uniform* (adj.)—not varying; similar in appearance, pattern, or color.

99. The correct answer is (D).
IMPROMPTU (adj.)—on the spur of the moment; improvised; extemporaneous. *Rehearsed* (adj.)—practiced beforehand.

100. The correct answer is (C).
WHIMSICAL (adj.)—capricious; impulsive. *Steadfast* (adj.)—immovable; not subject to change.

Chapter 7: Quantitative Ability

The PCAT Quantitative A̶b̶i̶l̶i̶t̶y̶ requires you to demonstrate your knowledge of and ability to work with basic arith̶m̶e̶t̶i̶c̶ etry. You will encounter word problems and also equations to simplify and ̶v̶i̶e̶w all of the relevant topics ahead of time in order to work as quickly as ̶i̶n̶volving units, it is prudent to write down the units along with the values ̶final calculated result has the correct units (e.g. grams, centimeters, and ̶ch of the three question types.

̶M̶EMBER

̶f fractions, decimal numbers, and percents using the
̶implemented with parentheses and various brackets
̶ the rules governing use of exponents (powers and
̶hms; knowledge of the metric system of measure

̶ulas given specific values for the variables
̶riptions into formulas
̶simultaneous equations, usually two equations in two unknowns

d) Obtaining the equation for a straight line (two-point method and slope-intercept method)

e) Calculation of the distance between two points given their x and y coordinates

f) Solving quadratic equations by factoring and by application of the Pythagorean Theorem

g) Solution by proportions for word problems

h) Determination of average, median, and mode

i) Solving simple probability theory problems

3) Geometry

a) Relationships between lines and angles

b) The types and sub-types of polygons, circles, cubes, cylinders, and spheres

c) Formulas for area of common objects, such as triangles, squares, rect-angles, and circles

d) Volume of cubes, cylinders, and spheres

Answer Sheet

Chapter 7: Quantitative Ability

1. Ⓐ Ⓑ Ⓒ Ⓓ   21. Ⓐ Ⓑ Ⓒ Ⓓ   41. Ⓐ Ⓑ Ⓒ Ⓓ   61. Ⓐ Ⓑ Ⓒ Ⓓ   81. Ⓐ Ⓑ Ⓒ Ⓓ

2. Ⓐ Ⓑ Ⓒ Ⓓ   22. Ⓐ Ⓑ Ⓒ Ⓓ   42. Ⓐ Ⓑ Ⓒ Ⓓ   62. Ⓐ Ⓑ Ⓒ Ⓓ   82. Ⓐ Ⓑ Ⓒ Ⓓ

3. Ⓐ Ⓑ Ⓒ Ⓓ   23. Ⓐ Ⓑ Ⓒ Ⓓ   43. Ⓐ Ⓑ Ⓒ Ⓓ   63. Ⓐ Ⓑ Ⓒ Ⓓ   83. Ⓐ Ⓑ Ⓒ Ⓓ

4. Ⓐ Ⓑ Ⓒ Ⓓ   24. Ⓐ Ⓑ Ⓒ Ⓓ   44. Ⓐ Ⓑ Ⓒ Ⓓ   64. Ⓐ Ⓑ Ⓒ Ⓓ   84. Ⓐ Ⓑ Ⓒ Ⓓ

5. Ⓐ Ⓑ Ⓒ Ⓓ   25. Ⓐ Ⓑ Ⓒ Ⓓ   45. Ⓐ Ⓑ Ⓒ Ⓓ   65. Ⓐ Ⓑ Ⓒ Ⓓ   85. Ⓐ Ⓑ Ⓒ Ⓓ

6. Ⓐ Ⓑ Ⓒ Ⓓ   26. Ⓐ Ⓑ Ⓒ Ⓓ   46. Ⓐ Ⓑ Ⓒ Ⓓ   66. Ⓐ Ⓑ Ⓒ Ⓓ   86. Ⓐ Ⓑ Ⓒ Ⓓ

7. Ⓐ Ⓑ Ⓒ Ⓓ   27. Ⓐ Ⓑ Ⓒ Ⓓ   47. Ⓐ Ⓑ Ⓒ Ⓓ   67. Ⓐ Ⓑ Ⓒ Ⓓ   87. Ⓐ Ⓑ Ⓒ Ⓓ

8. Ⓐ Ⓑ Ⓒ Ⓓ   28. Ⓐ Ⓑ Ⓒ Ⓓ   48. Ⓐ Ⓑ Ⓒ Ⓓ   68. Ⓐ Ⓑ Ⓒ Ⓓ   88. Ⓐ Ⓑ Ⓒ Ⓓ

9. Ⓐ Ⓑ Ⓒ Ⓓ   29. Ⓐ Ⓑ Ⓒ Ⓓ   49. Ⓐ Ⓑ Ⓒ Ⓓ   69. Ⓐ Ⓑ Ⓒ Ⓓ   89. Ⓐ Ⓑ Ⓒ Ⓓ

10. Ⓐ Ⓑ Ⓒ Ⓓ   30. Ⓐ Ⓑ Ⓒ Ⓓ   50. Ⓐ Ⓑ Ⓒ Ⓓ   70. Ⓐ Ⓑ Ⓒ Ⓓ   90. Ⓐ Ⓑ Ⓒ Ⓓ

11. Ⓐ Ⓑ Ⓒ Ⓓ   31. Ⓐ Ⓑ Ⓒ Ⓓ   51. Ⓐ Ⓑ Ⓒ Ⓓ   71. Ⓐ Ⓑ Ⓒ Ⓓ   91. Ⓐ Ⓑ Ⓒ Ⓓ

12. Ⓐ Ⓑ Ⓒ Ⓓ   32. Ⓐ Ⓑ Ⓒ Ⓓ   52. Ⓐ Ⓑ Ⓒ Ⓓ   72. Ⓐ Ⓑ Ⓒ Ⓓ   92. Ⓐ Ⓑ Ⓒ Ⓓ

13. Ⓐ Ⓑ Ⓒ Ⓓ   33. Ⓐ Ⓑ Ⓒ Ⓓ   53. Ⓐ Ⓑ Ⓒ Ⓓ   73. Ⓐ Ⓑ Ⓒ Ⓓ   93. Ⓐ Ⓑ Ⓒ Ⓓ

14. Ⓐ Ⓑ Ⓒ Ⓓ   34. Ⓐ Ⓑ Ⓒ Ⓓ   54. Ⓐ Ⓑ Ⓒ Ⓓ   74. Ⓐ Ⓑ Ⓒ Ⓓ   94. Ⓐ Ⓑ Ⓒ Ⓓ

15. Ⓐ Ⓑ Ⓒ Ⓓ   35. Ⓐ Ⓑ Ⓒ Ⓓ   55. Ⓐ Ⓑ Ⓒ Ⓓ   75. Ⓐ Ⓑ Ⓒ Ⓓ   95. Ⓐ Ⓑ Ⓒ Ⓓ

16. Ⓐ Ⓑ Ⓒ Ⓓ   36. Ⓐ Ⓑ Ⓒ Ⓓ   56. Ⓐ Ⓑ Ⓒ Ⓓ   76. Ⓐ Ⓑ Ⓒ Ⓓ   96. Ⓐ Ⓑ Ⓒ Ⓓ

17. Ⓐ Ⓑ Ⓒ Ⓓ   37. Ⓐ Ⓑ Ⓒ Ⓓ   57. Ⓐ Ⓑ Ⓒ Ⓓ   77. Ⓐ Ⓑ Ⓒ Ⓓ   97. Ⓐ Ⓑ Ⓒ Ⓓ

18. Ⓐ Ⓑ Ⓒ Ⓓ   38. Ⓐ Ⓑ Ⓒ Ⓓ   58. Ⓐ Ⓑ Ⓒ Ⓓ   78. Ⓐ Ⓑ Ⓒ Ⓓ   98. Ⓐ Ⓑ Ⓒ Ⓓ

19. Ⓐ Ⓑ Ⓒ Ⓓ   39. Ⓐ Ⓑ Ⓒ Ⓓ   59. Ⓐ Ⓑ Ⓒ Ⓓ   79. Ⓐ Ⓑ Ⓒ Ⓓ   99. Ⓐ Ⓑ Ⓒ Ⓓ

20. Ⓐ Ⓑ Ⓒ Ⓓ   40. Ⓐ Ⓑ Ⓒ Ⓓ   60. Ⓐ Ⓑ Ⓒ Ⓓ   80. Ⓐ Ⓑ Ⓒ Ⓓ   100. Ⓐ Ⓑ Ⓒ Ⓓ

Tear Here

Quantitative Ability Practice Questions

100 QUESTIONS—1 HOUR, 10 MINUTES

Directions: Choose the best answer to each of the following questions.

1. $\dfrac{3}{8} + \dfrac{4}{5} =$

   (A) $\dfrac{95}{80}$

   (B) 1.2

   (C) $1\dfrac{7}{40}$

   (D) $\dfrac{12}{40}$

2. $0.25 + \dfrac{15}{16} =$

   (A) 1.08

   (B) $1\dfrac{3}{16}$

   (C) 3.75

   (D) $\dfrac{24}{16}$

3. $1.30 \times 236 =$
   (A) 3.068×10^2
   (B) $3{,}068 \times 10^1$
   (C) 283.2
   (D) 29.9×10^2

4. $\log(50 \times 2) =$
   (A) $(\log 50) \times (\log 2)$
   (B) $(\log 2) \times (10 \log 5)$
   (C) $\log 10$
   (D) $\log 2 + \log 50$

5. $\log 0.001 =$
   (A) 3
   (B) 100
   (C) -3
   (D) $\dfrac{1}{3}$

6. $\sqrt[3]{8} =$

   (A) 2^3

   (B) $\dfrac{8}{2}$

   (C) $8^{\frac{1}{3}}$

   (D) $8 \log 3$

7. $\log_{10} 1{,}000 =$
   (A) 10
   (B) 3
   (C) 100
   (D) 4

8. $1 \times 10^{-2} + 2.3 \times 10^{1} =$

   (A) 2.3×10^{2}

   (B) 24.0

   (C) 23.01

   (D) 23.1

---

9. $\frac{3}{16} =$

   (A) 25%

   (B) $\frac{9}{32}$

   (C) 18.75%

   (D) 33%

---

10. $\frac{(2.3g.)}{(10ml.)} =$

   (A) 2.3%

   (B) 0.23%

   (C) $23\% \frac{wt.}{vol.}$

   (D) $\frac{2.3}{100}$

---

11. How many liters of a 4% solution can be made from 24 g. of a drug?

   (A) 6 liters

   (B) 0.6 liter

   (C) 0.096 liter

   (D) 96 liters

---

12. How much 0.9% NaCl can be made from 1 liter of an 18% stock solution of NaCl?

   (A) 0.05 liter

   (B) 5.0 liters

   (C) 2.0 liters

   (D) 20 liters

---

13. What is the percentage of ethanol in a mixture composed of 5 liters of 25%, 2 liters of 50%, and 0.5 liter of 10% ethanol?

   (A) 11.3%

   (B) 50%

   (C) 30.7%

   (D) 22%

---

14. $\log \sqrt{25} =$

   (A) $\frac{1}{2}\log 25$

   (B) $\log 25^{\frac{1}{2}}$

   (C) $\log 5$

   (D) All of the above

---

15. $\log 25^{2} =$

   (A) $\log 50$

   (B) 5

   (C) $\log 5$

   (D) $2 \times \log 25$

---

16. If 1 kg. equals 2.2 lbs., how many grams are in 1 lb.?

   (A) 454.5 g.

   (B) 2,200 g.

   (C) 97.8 g.

   (D) 1,200 g.

---

17. Subtract 283 ml. from 1 liter.

   (A) 217 ml.

   (B) 9,717 ml.

   (C) 717 ml.

   (D) None of the above

18. If 15.43 grains are in 1 g., how many milligrams equals 1 grain?

(A) 0.065 mg.

(B) 984.6 mg.

(C) 84.57 mg.

(D) 64.81 mg.

---

19. $\sqrt[3]{3^6} + \sqrt{2^2} =$

(A) 7

(B) 11

(C) 36

(D) None of the above

---

20. $\left(\dfrac{2}{3}\right)^2 + 2^{-3} =$

(A) $\dfrac{41}{72}$

(B) $\dfrac{4}{48}$

(C) $\dfrac{2}{24}$

(D) $\dfrac{2}{3}$

---

21. $10^0 + 10^1 + 10^{-1} =$

(A) 10.1

(B) 101

(C) 11.1

(D) 1.1

---

22. If $9\,(x°C) = 5(y°F) - 160$, what is 79°F in degrees centigrade?

(A) 23.5°C

(B) 87.1°C

(C) 26.1°C

(D) 174.2°C

---

23. What is –10°C in degrees Fahrenheit?

(A) 50°F

(B) 14°F

(C) –12.2°F

(D) –10°F

---

24. If the temperature dropped from 72°F to 65°F, by how many degrees centigrade did the temperature change?

(A) 7°C

(B) 13.9°C

(C) 44.6°C

(D) 3.9°C

---

25. What weight of a particular substance is needed to produce 200 ml. of a 1:10,000 solution?

(A) 1 g.

(B) 200 mg.

(C) 0.02 g.

(D) 2 mg.

Questions 26-30 refer to the following graph.

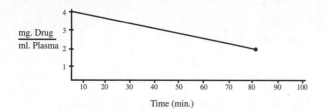

Time (min.)

26. At 20 minutes, how much drug remained in the plasma?
   (A)   2 mg./ml.
   (B)   There was no change.
   (C)   3.5 mg./ml.
   (D)   It cannot be determined.

27. At what rate is the drug disappearing from the plasma?
   (A)   2 mg./ml. plasma per 60 minutes
   (B)   4 mg./ml. plasma per 80 minutes
   (C)   1.5 mg./ml. plasma per hour
   (D)   None of the above

28. At 2 hours, what would be the concentration of drug in the plasma?
   (A)   0.5 mg./ml.
   (B)   1 mg./ml.
   (C)   No drug will remain.
   (D)   None of the above

29. If the initial drug concentration had been 8 mg./ml. and the rate of disappearance stayed the same, what would have been the drug concentration at 80 minutes?
   (A)   6 mg./ml.
   (B)   4 mg./ml.
   (C)   2 mg./ml.
   (D)   None of the above

30. How long would it take the drug concentration to reach 0 mg./ml. if the initial concentration was 4 mg./ml.?
   (A)   2 hours
   (B)   200 minutes
   (C)   160 minutes
   (D)   150 minutes

For Questions 31 and 32, find all positive *integers* satisfying the inequality.

31. $4 < 3x - 2 \leq 10$
   (A)   5, 6, 7, 8, 9, 10
   (B)   1, 2, 3
   (C)   3, 4
   (D)   None of the above

32. $\frac{7}{x} > 2$, with $x \neq 0$
   (A)   7
   (B)   1, 2, 3
   (C)   2, 7
   (D)   None of the above

33. $\left| -5 \right| - \left| -2 \right| =$
   (A)   -3
   (B)   7
   (C)   3
   (D)   -7

34. $|8| - |14| =$

    (A)   6

    (B)   -6

    (C)   22

    (D)   None of the above

---

35. Solve $|5x + 4| = -3$ for x.

    (A) $\dfrac{7}{5}$

    (B) $\dfrac{1}{5}$

    (C)   2

    (D)   None of the above

> **Questions 36–38 refer to the following diagram.**

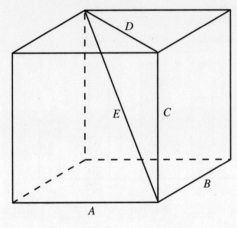

$A = B = C$ $A = 2$ in.

36. What is the length of line D?

    (A)   2 in.

    (B) $\sqrt{8}$ in.

    (C)   4 in.

    (D) $\sqrt{5}$ in.

37. What is the area encompassed by lines C, D, and E?

    (A) $\sqrt{8}$ in.²

    (B) $2\sqrt{3}$ in.²

    (C)   2 in.²

    (D)   4 in.²

38. What is the total surface area of the cube?

    (A)   24 in.²

    (B)   16 in.²

    (C)   12 in.²

    (D)   32 in.²

> **Questions 39–42 refer to the following diagram.**

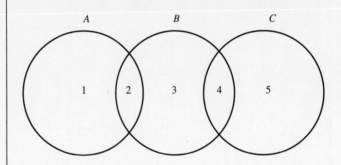

39. The subset _A or B_ encompasses area(s)

    (A)   1 and 3.

    (B)   2 only.

    (C)   1, 2, and 3.

    (D)   1, 2, 3, and 4.

---

40. The subset _A and B_ encompasses area(s)

    (A)   1 and 3.

    (B)   2 only.

    (C)   1, 2, and 3.

    (D)   1, 2, 3, and 4.

41. The subset _A or C, but not B_ encompasses area(s)

  (A) 1 and 5.

  (B) 1, 2, 4, and 5.

  (C) 2 and 4.

  (D) 1, 4, and 5.

42. The subset _B only_ encompasses area(s)

  (A) 1 and 3.

  (B) 2, 3, and 4.

  (C) 2 and 4.

  (D) 3 only.

Questions 43–45 refer to the following diagrams.

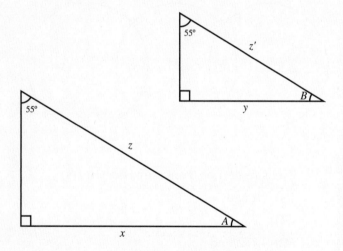

43. If $x = 2y$, what is the ratio of the areas of the two triangles ($x:y$) above?

  (A) 2:1

  (B) 4:1

  (C) 1:2

  (D) $\sqrt{2}$:1

44. How many degrees are there in angle A?

  (A) 60°

  (B) 45°

  (C) 90°

  (D) 35°

45. If $x = 3y$ and $z = 5$, what is z'?

  (A) $\sqrt{5}$

  (B) 3

  (C) $\dfrac{3}{5}$

  (D) $1\dfrac{2}{3}$

Questions 46 and 47 refer to the following graph.

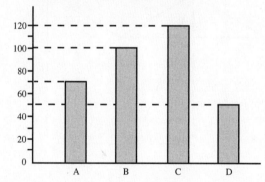

Percentage of drug assayed as compared to the manufacturer's declared amount.

46. If a minimum of 90% of the declared amount of active drug is required by law, which drugs may be used?

  (A) C only

  (B) B and C

  (C) A, B, and C

  (D) None of the above

47. If the amount of drug declared by the manufacturer was 200 mg., how much drug was present in the drug samples accepted in the previous question?

(A) 200 mg.

(B) 100 and 120 mg.

(C) 200 and 240 mg.

(D) None of the above

> Questions 48–50 refer to the following graph.

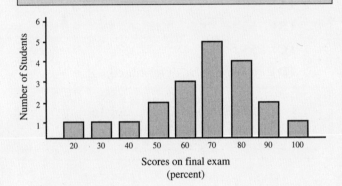

48. What is the mean percent score for the final exam?

(A) 70%

(B) 60%

(C) 66%

(D) 80%

49. What is the modal score?

(A) 70%

(B) 60%

(C) 66%

(D) 80%

50. What is the median score?

(A) 70%

(B) 60%

(C) 66%

(D) 80%

51. If 50 tablets contain 0.625 g. of active ingredient, how many tablets can be prepared from 31.25 g. of ingredient?

(A) 2,500 tablets

(B) 25 tablets

(C) 625 tablets

(D) 100 tablets

52. The adult (weight, 150 lbs.) dose of a drug is 70 µg. Approximately what is the dose for a child weighing 44 lbs.?

(A) 200 µg.

(B) 20 µg.

(C) 3 µg.

(D) None of the above

53. If $x = \frac{1}{y}$, what happens to y when x is increased to $2x$?

(A) y increases by a factor of 2

(B) y decreases by a factor of $\frac{1}{2}$

(C) There is no change in y

(D) y increases by a factor of 4

54. If $x = 2y$, what happens to y when x is increased to $2x$?

(A) y increases by a factor of 2

(B) y decreases by a factor of $\frac{1}{2}$

(C) There is no change in y

(D) y increases by a factor of 4

55. A quantity of drug weighing 24 g. is divided into 16 equal parts. How much does each part weigh?

   (A) 150 mg.
   (B) 2,666 mg.
   (C) 0.150 g.
   (D) 1,500 mg.

56. If there may be a 10% error in the weight of a tablet, what is the range of acceptable tablet weights when a tablet of 150 g. is desired?

   (A) 135–150 g.
   (B) 140–160 g.
   (C) 130–170 g.
   (D) 135–165 g.

57. If there are 65 mg. of elemental iron in 325 mg. of ferrous sulfate, what percentage of the tablet weight is due to the iron?

   (A) 20%
   (B) 2%
   (C) 5%
   (D) 50%

58. A compound has a maximal solubility of 50 mg./ml. How much is needed to make a 1 liter solution at the maximal concentration?

   (A) 5,000 mg.
   (B) 20 g.
   (C) 1,000 mg.
   (D) 50 g.

59. If a graduated cylinder is marked in 5-ml. intervals, what is the smallest volume that can be measured with a 10% error?

   (A) 5 ml.
   (B) 50 ml.
   (C) 100 ml.
   (D) 10 ml.

60. Give the average of the following to the nearest whole number: 61, 50, 100, 50.

   (A) 50
   (B) 65
   (C) 55
   (D) It cannot be determined.

Questions 61–63 refer to the following graph.

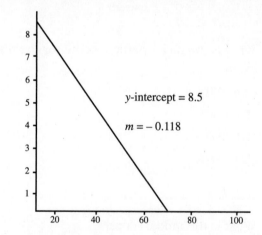

y-intercept = 8.5

$m = -0.118$

61. What is the equation for the line?

   (A) $y = 8.5 + 0.118x$
   (B) $8.5y = 0.118x$
   (C) $y = -0.118x + 8.5$
   (D) $y = -\dfrac{0.118x}{8.5}$

62. If y equals 6, what is the value of x to the nearest whole number?

   (A) 21
   (B) 40
   (C) 123
   (D) 10

63. If $x = 0$, what is the value of y?

   (A) 0.0
   (B) 0.118
   (C) 8.5
   (D) None of the above

Questions 64–66 refer to the following diagram.

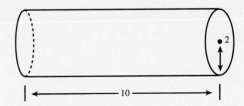

64. What is the volume of the cylinder ($\pi \cong 3.14$)?

   (A) 987 cubic units
   (B) 314 cubic units
   (C) 126 cubic units
   (D) 63 cubic units

65. What is the lateral surface area of the cylinder?

   (A) 987 square units
   (B) 314 square units
   (C) 126 square units
   (D) 63 square units

66. What is the total surface area of the cylinder?

   (A) 314 square units
   (B) 151 square units
   (C) 126 square units
   (D) 135 square units

67. What is the area of the trapezoid when $a = 4$, $b = 2$, and $h = 1$?

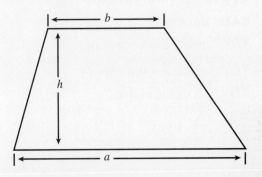

   (A) 4 square units
   (B) 3 square units
   (C) 6 square units
   (D) 8 square units

68. What is the area of the parallelogram when $b = 5$ and $h = 2$?

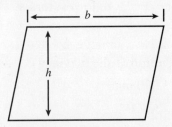

   (A) 5 square units
   (B) 20 square units
   (C) 10 square units
   (D) 2.5 square units

69. If $y = 3a + b$ and $x = 3b + a$, find y in terms of x and b.

(A) $3b + 8x$

(B) $3b - 8x$

(C) $3x - 8b$

(D) $3x + 8b$

70. Given the equation $y = mx + c$, a linear plot of y versus x will yield a(n)

(A) slope of m.

(B) ordinate intercept of $\dfrac{1}{c}$.

(C) abscissa intercept of c.

(D) All of the above

71. $\dfrac{(7 \div 3)}{(21 \div 3)} =$

(A) $\dfrac{7}{21}$

(B) $\dfrac{1}{3}$

(C) 0.33

(D) All of the above

72. Reduce $\dfrac{72}{2,880}$ to lowest terms.

(A) $\dfrac{1}{120}$

(B) $\dfrac{1}{124}$

(C) $\dfrac{1}{52}$

(D) $\dfrac{1}{40}$

73. A prescription calls for 7.5 mg. of a drug. How many tablets containing 0.25 mg. of the drug are required?

(A) 30

(B) 31

(C) 15

(D) 17

74. Add $\dfrac{3}{4}$ mg., 0.25 mg., $\dfrac{2}{5}$ mg., and 2.75 mg.

(A) 5.0 mg.

(B) 4.0 mg.

(C) 4.15 mg.

(D) 5.15 mg.

75. Add 0.75 mg., 50 g., and .5 kg.

(A) 550.00075 g.

(B) 500.75 g.

(C) 0.5575 kg.

(D) 500,575 mg.

76. $3\dfrac{1}{8}$ is the same as

(A) $\dfrac{75}{36}$

(B) $\dfrac{100}{32}$

(C) $\dfrac{125}{32}$

(D) $\dfrac{125}{36}$

77. If 60 mg. = 1 grain, then 10% of 360 mg. =

    (A) 6 grain

    (B) 0.6 grain

    (C) 0.06 grain

    (D) 60 grain

---

78. $2\sqrt{36} + \dfrac{4\sqrt{28}}{3\sqrt{7}} =$

    (A) $14\sqrt{7}$

    (B) $12\dfrac{2}{3}$

    (C) $13\sqrt{7}$

    (D) $14\dfrac{2}{3}$

---

79. If $A = e^a$, then $1 + A =$

    (A) $1 + e^a$

    (B) e^a

    (C) $\dfrac{1}{e^a}$

    (D) $\ln e^a$

---

80. $7.7 \times 10^0 =$

    (A) 0

    (B) 0.77

    (C) 7.7

    (D) 77

---

81. 1,000,000 can also be expressed as

    (A) $1 \times 10^6 \times 10^1$

    (B) $1 \times 10^3 \times 10^{-3}$

    (C) $1 \times 10^3 \times 10^3$

    (D) $1 \times 10^6 \times 10^{-3}$

---

82. $\sqrt{144 \times 10^4} =$

    (A) 2,400

    (B) 800

    (C) 1,600

    (D) 1,200

---

83. If 1 kg = 2.2 lbs., add the following and express the answer in kilograms: 132 lbs., 11 lbs., and 44 lbs.

    (A) 85 kg.

    (B) 88 kg.

    (C) 98 kg.

    (D) 58 kg.

---

84. $\left(\dfrac{3}{4}\right)^2 + 3^2 + \sqrt{\dfrac{49}{256}} =$

    (A) 27

    (B) 10

    (C) 29

    (D) 30

---

85. A given line has a slope of −2 and a y-intercept $(0, \sqrt{2})$. It can be expressed as the linear equation

    (A) $y = -2x.$

    (B) $y = \sqrt{2} + 2x.$

    (C) $y = -2x + \sqrt{2}.$

    (D) $y = 2x.$

86. Find the value of $\dfrac{250{,}000 \times 0.018}{0.15}$.

   (A) 300,000

   (B) 275,000

   (C) 37,000

   (D) 30,000

---

87. What is x if $x^{-3} = \dfrac{1}{27}$?

   (A) 3

   (B) $\dfrac{1}{3}$

   (C) 0.6

   (D) 9

---

88. What is I?

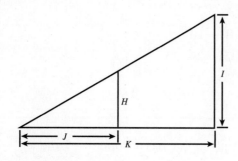

   (A) $\dfrac{KH}{J}$

   (B) $\dfrac{JH}{K}$

   (C) $\dfrac{JK}{H}$

   (D) None of the above

> **Questions 89–93 refer to the following statement:**

A compound is composed (by weight) of drug A, 20%; drug B, 5%; and drug C, 75%.

89. What amount of drug A is required to make 500 g. of the compound?

   (A) 100 g.

   (B) 125 g.

   (C) 375 g.

   (D) 400 g.

---

90. What amount of drugs A and B is needed to make 500 g. of the compound?

   (A) 100 g.

   (B) 125 g.

   (C) 375 g.

   (D) 400 g.

---

91. What amount of drugs B and C is needed to make 500 g. of the compound?

   (A) 100 g.

   (B) 125 g.

   (C) 375 g.

   (D) 400 g.

---

92. What amount of drugs A, B, and C is needed to make 100 g. of the compound?

   (A) 100 g.

   (B) 125 g.

   (C) 375 g.

   (D) 400 g.

93. What are the ratios A:B:C as indicated in the formula?

- **(A)** 4:15:1
- **(B)** 4:1:15
- **(C)** 15:1:4
- **(D)** None of the above

---

94. Given that $\dfrac{B-p}{q} = \dfrac{\dfrac{g_a}{M_{-a}}}{\dfrac{g_b}{M_b}}$, find g_b.

- **(A)** $\dfrac{B-p}{q}\dfrac{M_a M_b}{g_a}$

- **(B)** $\dfrac{p-B}{q}\dfrac{M_b g_a}{M_a}$

- **(C)** $\dfrac{q}{B-p} M_b M_a M_a$

- **(D)** $\dfrac{q}{B-p}\dfrac{M_b g_a}{M_a}$

95. Consider the following:

Equation 1 $y = 3x + 4$
Equation 2 $y = 3x - 4$

Which best describes equations 1 and 2, respectively?

- **(A)** Slope of +4, y-intercept of +3, slope of -4, and y-intercept of -3
- **(B)** x-intercept of +3, slope of +4, x-intercept of -3, and slope of -4
- **(C)** y-intercept of +3, slope of +4, y-intercept of -3, and slope of -4
- **(D)** Slope of +3, y-intercept of +4, slope of +3, and y-intercept of -4

---

96. For the following equations, solve for a and b:

$30 = a + 3b - 70$ and $3a + 5b = 100$

- **(A)** $a = -50, b = 50$
- **(B)** $a = 5, b = -5$
- **(C)** $a = -5, b = 5$
- **(D)** $a = 50, b = -50$

---

97. How much medicine would provide a patient with 2 tablespoons twice a day for 10 days? (1 tablespoon = 15 ml.)

- **(A)** 300 ml.
- **(B)** 600 ml.
- **(C)** 450 ml.
- **(D)** 900 ml.

98. If 0.060 of a substance is employed in preparing 125 tablets, how much substance is contained in each tablet?

(A) 390 μg.

(B) 420 μg.

(C) 450 μg.

(D) 480 μg.

---

99. A patient's eye patch measures 12.70 cm. across. You have a tape measure in inches. How many inches does the eye patch measure? (1 in. = 2.54 cm.)

(A) 17 in.

(B) 10 in.

(C) 5 in.

(D) 3 in.

100. $\left(\dfrac{1}{120} \div \dfrac{1}{150} \right) \times 50 =$

(A) $62\dfrac{1}{2}$

(B) 40

(C) $50\dfrac{1}{2}$

(D) 25

ANSWER KEY

Quantitative Ability				
1. C	21. C	41. A	61. C	81. C
2. B	22. C	42. D	62. A	82. D
3. A	23. B	43. B	63. C	83. A
4. D	24. D	44. D	64. C	84. B
5. C	25. C	45. D	65. C	85. C
6. C	26. C	46. B	66. B	86. D
7. B	27. C	47. C	67. B	87. A
8. C	28. B	48. C	68. C	88. A
9. C	29. A	49. A	69. C	89. A
10. C	30. C	50. A	70. A	90. B
11. B	31. C	51. A	71. D	91. D
12. D	32. B	52. B	72. D	92. A
13. C	33. C	53. B	73. A	93. B
14. C	34. A	54. A	74. C	94. D
15. D	35. D	55. D	75. A	95. D
16. A	36. B	56. D	76. B	96. A
17. C	37. A	57. A	77. B	97. B
18. D	38. A	58. D	78. D	98. D
19. B	39. D	59. B	79. A	99. C
20. A	40. B	60. B	80. C	100. A

EXPLANATORY ANSWERS

1. **The correct answer is (C).**

   To add or subtract fractions, convert to equivalent fractions with the same least common denominator (LCD):

   $$\frac{3}{8} + \frac{4}{5} = \frac{3 \times 5}{8 \times 5} + \frac{4 \times 8}{5 \times 8}$$
   $$= \frac{15}{40} + \frac{32}{40}$$
   $$= \frac{47}{40}$$
   $$= 1\frac{7}{40}$$

2. **The correct answer is (B).**

   To add or subtract arithmetic fractions and decimal fractions, convert to a common base:

   $$0.25 + \frac{15}{16} = \frac{4}{16} + \frac{15}{16}$$
   $$= \frac{19}{16}$$
   $$= 1\frac{3}{16}$$

   or

   $$0.25 + \frac{15}{16} = 0.25 + 0.9375$$
   $$= 1.1875$$

3. **The correct answer is (A).**

   The following relations may be used when dealing with scientific notation:

   $$10^0 = 1$$
   $$10^{-A} = \frac{1}{10^A}$$
   $$10^{A+B} = 10^A \times 10^B$$
   $$\frac{10^A}{10^B} = 10^{A-B}$$
   $$\left(10^A\right)^B = 10^{AB}$$

Since

$$1.30 = 1.30 \times 10^0$$

and

$$236 = 2.36 \times 10^2$$

we have

$$(1.30 \times 10^0) \times (2.36 \times 10^2) = 3.068 \times 10^{0+2}$$
$$= 3.068 \times 10^2$$

4. **The correct answer is (D).**

   The log of a product equals the sum of the logs of the component numbers:

   $$\log (50 \times 2) = \log 50 + \log 2 = \log 2 + \log 50$$

5. **The correct answer is (C).**

   The logs of multiples of 10, for example, 1, 10, 0.1, are integers:

$10^2 = 100$	$\log 100 = 2$
$10^1 = 10$	$\log 10 = 1$
$10^0 = 1$	$\log 1 = 0$
$10^{-1} = 0.1$	$\log 0.1 = -1$
$10^{-2} = 0.01$	$\log 0.01 = -2$
$10^{-3} = 0.001$	$\log 0.001 = -3$

6. **The correct answer is (C).**

   The root of a power is found by dividing the exponent of the power of the index of the root (see the law of exponents in Answer 19):

   $$\sqrt[3]{8}$$

   8 is the power

   1 is the exponent

   3 is the root

   $$= 8^{\frac{1}{3}}$$

7. **The correct answer is (B).**

   The log of a number is the exponent of the power to which a given base must be raised in order to equal that number; that is, if

   $$y = a^x$$

   then

   $$\log_a y = x$$

   Therefore,

   $$\log_{10} 1,000 = 3$$

   or base 10 raised to the third power equals 1,000.

8. **The correct answer is (C).**

When adding or subtracting in scientific notation, convert to the same exponent, then add the products; the exponent will remain constant:

$$1 \times 10^{-2} = 0.01 \times 10^{0}$$

and

$$2.3 \times 10^{1} = 23 \times 10^{0}$$

So,

$$(0.01 \times 10^{0}) + (23 \times 10^{0}) = 23.01 \times 10^{0}$$
$$= 23.01$$

9. **The correct answer is (C).**

Percent, written as %, means per hundred. It is a type of ratio and thus has no units. To express a fraction as a percentage, set 100 as the denominator and multiply by 100%:

$$\frac{3}{16} \times 100\% = 0.1875 \times 100\%$$

$$= 18.75\%$$

10. **The correct answer is (C).**

Weight-per-volume measurements are often expressed as percentages. To calculate the percent weight per volume, convert the fraction to a percentage, that is, with a denominator of 100, times 100%:

$$\frac{2.3 \text{ g.}}{10 \text{ ml.}} = \frac{23 \text{ g.}}{100 \text{ ml.}}$$

and

$$\frac{23 \text{ g.}}{100 \text{ ml.}} \times 100\% = 23\% \frac{\text{wt.}}{\text{vol.}}$$

11. **The correct answer is (B).**

This problem involves the use of two ratios set equal to one another to form an equation known as a proportion. To solve a proportion, only one number may be unknown, which will be called x. To solve, rearrange the equation such that x remains alone. Given $A:B = C:D$, the following rules may be used:

1. The product of the means equals the product of the extremes: $B \times C = A \times D$.

2. The product of the means divided by one extreme gives the other extreme:

$$\frac{BC}{A} = D$$

3. The product of the extremes divided by one mean gives the other mean:

$$\frac{AD}{B} = C$$

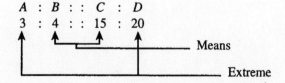

Therefore,

$$4\% \text{ solution} = \frac{4 \text{ g.}}{100 \text{ ml.}} \text{ (as explained in Answer 10) and}$$

x = number of liters in which 24 g. will be dissolved.

(*Note:* 1,000 ml. = 1 liter.)

Since

$$4 \text{ g.} : 100 \text{ ml.} : : 24 \text{ g.} : x \text{ ml.}$$

then

$$\frac{4 \text{ g.}}{100 \text{ ml.}} = \frac{24 \text{ g.}}{x}$$

$$x = \frac{24 \text{ g.} \times 100 \text{ ml.}}{4 \text{ g.}}$$

$$= 600 \text{ ml. or } 0.6 \text{ liter}$$

12. **The correct answer is (D).**

This problem is similar to that of Question 11 in that a proportionality is needed to solve the problem. First determine the total number of grams of NaCl that will be used to make the 0.9% solution:

$$18\% = \frac{18 \text{ g.}}{100 \text{ ml.}} \times 1,000 \text{ ml.}$$

$$= 180 \text{ g.}$$

This quantity will be diluted with the final total volume, the unknown x, which should result in a 0.9% solution:

$$0.9\% = \frac{0.9 \text{ g.}}{100 \text{ ml.}}$$

and

$$\frac{0.9\%}{100 \text{ ml.}} = \frac{180 \text{ g.}}{x \text{ ml.}}$$

So,

$$x \text{ ml.} = \frac{180 \text{ g.} \times 100 \text{ ml.}}{0.9 \text{ g.}}$$

$$= 20,000 \text{ ml.}$$

$$= 20 \text{ liters}$$

13. The correct answer is (C).

When one mixes different strengths, the units and types of percent (wt./wt., wt./vol., vol./vol.) must be kept constant. Determine the total amount of ethanol in all solutions and the total amount of solution, assuming additivity of volumes on mixing. Then, convert to the desired final ration:

$$25\% \times 5,000 \text{ ml.} = 1,250 \text{ ml.}$$

$$50\% \times 2,000 \text{ ml.} = 1,000 \text{ ml.}$$

$$10\% \times \frac{50 \text{ ml.}}{7,500 \text{ ml.}} = \frac{50 \text{ ml.}}{2,300 \text{ ml.}} \text{ ethanol}$$

So

$$\frac{2,300 \text{ ml of ethanol}}{7,500 \text{ ml of solution}} = 0.3067 \cong 30.7\%$$

14. The correct answer is (C).

The laws of logarithms are derived from the laws of exponents (see Answer 19). The most commonly used base is 10, although any base may be used.

$$\log (ab) = \log a + \log b$$

$$\log \left(\frac{a}{b}\right) = \log a - \log b$$

$$\log a^n = n \times \log a$$

$$\log a^{\frac{1}{n}} = \log \sqrt[n]{a} = \left(\frac{1}{n}\right) \log a$$

Therefore,

$$\log \sqrt{25} = \frac{1}{2} \log 25 = \frac{(\log 25)}{2}$$

$$= \log 25^{\frac{1}{2}}$$

$$= \log 5$$

15. The correct answer is (D).

From previous answers,

$$\log a^n = n \times \log a$$

$$\log 25^2 = 2 \times \log 25$$

16. **The correct answer is (A).**

    This problem involves ratios. First convert the common units:

    $$1 \text{ kg.} = 1{,}000 \text{ g.}$$

    Then set up the proportionality:

    $$\frac{1 \text{ kg.}}{2.2 \text{ lbs.}} = \frac{x}{1 \text{ lb.}}$$

    $$\frac{1{,}000 \text{ g.} \times \left(1 \text{ lb.}\right)}{2.2 \text{ lbs.}} = x$$

    $$454.5 \text{ g.} = x$$

17. **The correct answer is (C).**

    Whenever mathematical procedures are used, all the units must be the same. Therefore,

    $$1 \text{ liter} = 1{,}000 \text{ ml.}$$

    and

    $$1{,}000 \text{ ml.} - 283 \text{ ml.} = 717 \text{ ml.}$$

18. **The correct answer is (D).**

    (See Answers 11 and 16.)

    $$\text{Since } 1 \text{ g.} = 1{,}000 \text{ mg.}$$

    we have

    $$\frac{15.43 \text{ grains}}{1{,}000 \text{ mg.}} = \frac{1 \text{ grain}}{x \text{ mg.}}$$

    $$x \text{ mg.} = \frac{1 \text{ grain} \times 1{,}000 \text{ mg.}}{15.43 \text{ grains}}$$

    $$x = 64.81 \text{ mg.}$$

19. **The correct answer is (B).**

First simplify the numbers (see Answer 6); then use the law of exponents:

1. The product of two or more powers of the *same base* is the base with an exponent equal to the *sum of all the exponents*:

$$4^3 \times 4^{10} = 4^{10+3} = 4^{13}$$

2. The quotient of two powers with the *same base* is the base with an exponent equal to the *exponent of the numerator minus that of the denominator*:

$$\frac{3^8}{3^2} = 3^{8-2} = 3^6$$

3. The power of a power is found by *multiplying the exponents*:

$$(2^4)^3 = 2^{4 \times 3} = 2^{12}$$

4. The power of a product equals the *product of the powers* of the factors:

$$(2 \times 3 \times 4)^2 = 2^2 \times 3^2 \times 4^2$$

5. The root of a power is found by *dividing the exponent of the power by the index of the root*:

$$\sqrt[3]{8^6} = 8^{\frac{6}{3}} = 8^2$$

6. The power of a fraction equals the *power of the numerator divided by the power of the denominator*:

$$\left(\frac{2}{3}\right)^2 = \frac{2^2}{3^2}$$

7. A number with a *negative* exponent equals 1 divided by the number with a positive exponent:

$$12^{-2} = \frac{1}{12^2}$$

8. Any number other than 0 with exponent 0 equals 1:

$$10^0 = 1, \ 4^0 = 1, \ 1^0 = 1$$

Therefore, for Question 19 we have $\sqrt[3]{3^6} = 3^{\frac{6}{3}} = 3^2$ and $\sqrt{2^2} = 2^{\frac{2}{2}} = 2^1 = 2$ so,

$$3^2 + 2 = (3 \times 3) + 2$$

$$3^2 + 2 = 11$$

20. The correct answer is (A).

Making the appropriate conversion to the least common denominator, we have

$$\left(\frac{2}{3}\right)^2 + 2^{-3} = \frac{2^2}{3^2} + \frac{1}{2^3}$$

$$= \frac{4}{9} + \frac{1}{8}$$

$$= \frac{4 \times 8}{9 \times 8} + \frac{9 \times 1}{9 \times 8}$$

$$= \frac{32}{72} + \frac{9}{72}$$

$$= \frac{41}{72}$$

21. The correct answer is (C).

$$10^0 = 1$$

$$10^1 = 10$$

$$\underline{10^{-1} = 0.1}$$

$$11.1$$

22. The correct answer is (C).

In problems involving formulas, rearrange the formula until the unknown term is expressed by all the other terms. Therefore, if the temperature in degrees centigrade is unknown, rearrange the formula as follows:

$$9(x°C) \;=\; 5(y°F) - 160$$

$$x°C \;=\; \frac{5}{9}(y°F) - \frac{160}{9}$$

$$=\; \frac{5 \times 79}{9} - 17.78$$

$$=\; 26.1$$

23. The correct answer is (B).

Rearrange to solve for the temperature in degrees Fahrenheit, as explained above:

$$9(x°C) \;=\; 5(y°F) - 160$$

$$5(x°F) \;=\; 9(x°C) + 160$$

$$x°F \;=\; \frac{9}{5}(x°C) + \frac{160}{5}$$

$$=\; \frac{9° \times \left(\pm 10°\right)}{5°} + 32°$$

$$=\; -18° + 32°$$

$$=\; 14°F$$

24. The correct answer is (D).

This problem may be approached by determining the respective temperatures in degrees centigrade and then computing the difference.

From

$$x°C = \frac{5(y°F) - 160}{9}$$

we have

$$x°C = \frac{5(72) - 160}{9}, \qquad x'°C = \frac{5(65) - 160}{9}$$

$$x°C = 22.22, \qquad x'°C \cong 18.33$$

So,

$$22.22 - 18.33 \cong 3.88 \qquad 3.9°C$$

Alternately, as one degree Fahrenheit is $\frac{9}{5}$ of a degree on the centigrade scale, the problem may be solved by multiplying the differences in degrees Fahrenheit by $\frac{5}{9}$.

$$72°F - 65°F = 7°F$$

$$7°F \times \frac{5}{9} = \frac{35}{9} = 3.88°C$$

You cannot directly substitute the 7°F into the temperature conversion equation as originally given, since that equation converts the 7°F to the corresponding temperature in degrees centigrade. That is, 7°F equals −13.8°C.

25. The correct answer is (C).

This is a proportionality problem. Assume a weight-volume relationship:

$$1 : 10,000 :: x : 200 :$$

$$\frac{1 \text{ g.}}{10,000 \text{ ml.}} = \frac{x \text{ g.}}{200 \text{ ml.}}$$

$$x \text{ g.} = \frac{(1 \text{ g.}) \times (200 \text{ ml.})}{10,000 \text{ ml.}}$$

$$= 0.02 \text{ g.}$$

26. The correct answer is (C).

When x is known, y may be found by drawing a line up from the x-axis, parallel to the y-axis, until the line of the graph is intersected. A line is then drawn from this point perpendicular to the y-axis until it is intersected. This is the value of y for a given x.

27.   The correct answer is (C).

The rate of drug disappearance is the change in y (mg. drug/ml. plasma) over a range of x (time). This is equal to the slope:

$$\frac{y_2 - y_1}{x_2 - x_1} = m$$

Therefore, to determine the rate (slope), any two y-values and corresponding x-values are needed: For example,

$$\text{time}_1 = 0 \text{ min.,} \qquad y_1 = \frac{\text{mg. drug}}{\text{ml. plasma}} = 4$$

$$\text{time}_2 = 80 \text{ min.,} \quad y_2 = \frac{\text{mg. drug}}{\text{ml. plasma}} = 2$$

Then,

$$\text{rate} = \frac{2-4}{80-0} = \frac{-2}{80} = \frac{-1}{40}$$

and

$$\frac{-1}{40} = \frac{-1 \text{ mg. / ml. plasma}}{40 \text{ min.}} = -1.5 \text{ mg./ml. plasma per hour}$$

Note: The negative sign indicates a decline, or falling y values, for increasing x values.

28.   The correct answer is (B).

To predict a y value for a given x, the slope m and the y-intercept b must be known so we can solve $y - mx + b$. From Answer 27,

$$m = \frac{-1.5 \text{ mg. / ml. plasma}}{1 \text{ hr.}}$$

and

$$b = 4 \text{ mg./ml. plasma}$$

$$x = 2 \text{ hrs.}$$

So,

$$y = (-1.5 \text{ mg./ml. per hour}) \times (2 \text{ hrs.}) + 4 \text{ mg./ml.}$$

$$= -3 \text{ mg./ml.} + 4 \text{ mg./ml.}$$

$$= 1 \text{ mg./ml.}$$

Remember to include the negative sign in the slope.

29. **The correct answer is (A).**

In this problem, the y-intercept has been changed to 8 mg./ml. and the time to 80 min. (1.33 hrs.). The problem is then solved as above:

$$y = mx + b$$

$$= (-1.5 \text{ mg./ml. per hour}) \times (1.33 \text{ hrs.}) + 8 \text{ mg./hr.}$$

$$= -1.995 + 8$$

$$\cong 6 \text{ mg./ml.}$$

30. **The correct answer is (C).**

This problem requires finding the value of x (time) when y (concentration) is zero. Again,

$$y \text{ is } mx + b$$

$$0 = (-1.5 \text{ mg./ml. per hour})x + 4 \text{ mg./ml.}$$

$$\frac{-4 \text{ mg./ml.}}{-1.5 \text{ mg./ml. per hour}} = x$$

$$2.66 \text{ hrs.} = x$$

$$160 \text{ min.} = x$$

31. **The correct answer is (C).**

An integer is any of the natural numbers, the negatives of the numbers and zero. To find the values for the inequalities, solve each of the inequalities separately; then delete all values *not* satisfying *both*:

$4 < 3x - 2 \le 10$	$3x - 2 \le 10$
$4 < 3x - 2$	$3x \le 10 + 2$
$4 + 2 < 3x$	$3x \le 12$
$\dfrac{6}{3} < x$	$x \le 4$
$2 < x$	

Therefore, all values greater than 2 may be accepted:
$3, 4, 5, \ldots, n$

Therefore, all values less than or equal to 4 will be accepted:
$4, 3, 2, 1, 0, -1, -2, \ldots, -n$

Integer values common to both inequalities are 3 and 4.

32. **The correct answer is (B).**

$$\frac{7}{x} > 2, \quad x \ne 0$$

$$7 > 2x$$

$$\frac{7}{2} > x$$

$$3.5 > x$$

x must be less than 3.5, or 3, 2, 1, 0, -1, -2..., but x cannot be 0; therefore 3, 2, 1 are common to both equations.

33. **The correct answer is (C).**

    The absolute value $|x|$ removes the sign of the number enclosed after all arithmetic functions enclosed have been completed, or $|-x| = x$.

    Therefore

    $$\left| -5 \right| - \left| -2 \right| = 5 - 2 = 3$$

34. **The correct answer is (A).**

    $$\left| 8 - 14 \right| = \left| -6 \right| = 6$$

35. **The correct answer is (D).**

    $$\left| 5x + 4 \right| = -3$$

    This problem cannot be solved, as there is no term whose absolute value will yield a negative result.

36. **The correct answer is (B).**

    As the figure is a cube, D is the hypotenuse of a right triangle with equal sides. From the Pythagorean Theorem, we have hypotenuse^2 = side^2 + side^2

    $$x^2 = 2^2 + 2^2$$
    $$x^2 = 4 + 4$$
    $$x^2 = 8$$
    $$x = \sqrt{8}$$

37. **The correct answer is (A).**

    In this example, lines C, D, and E form a right triangle with base D and side C (or base C and side D). If C is 2 in. (given condition) and D, from the previous example, is $\sqrt{8}$ in., then $\frac{1}{2}$ $\sqrt{8}$ (2) = $\sqrt{8}$ in.^{2} (The area of a triangle is equal to $\frac{1}{2}$ base × height.) E could also serve as a base, except, as E was unknown, it was easier to work with the sides already known.

38. **The correct answer is (A).**

    A cube has six faces: top, bottom, and four sides. If each face has a surface area of 2×2 in.^{2}, then the total area is

    $$\frac{\left(2 \text{ in.} \times 2 \text{ in.} \right)}{\text{face}} \times 6 \text{ faces} = 24 \text{ in.}^2$$

39. **The correct answer is (D).**

    The subset of *A or B* includes all subsets for *A* (1, 2) plus all subsets of *B* (2, 3, 4); that is, all cases in which the condition of *A or B* has been met will be accepted (1, 2, 3, 4).

40. **The correct answer is (B).**

    A subset *A and B* includes all cases in which *both* the conditions of subset *A* and subset *B* must be met (2 only).

41. **The correct answer is (A).**

    The subset *A or C* includes all cases satisfying the conditions of subset *A* (1, 2) plus those satisfying the conditions of *C* (4, 5). However, any cases also included in *B* must be excluded (2, 3, or 4), for the subset we are looking for is *A or C*, but not *B*. Therefore, only subsets 1 and 5 may be accepted.

42. **The correct answer is (D).**

    The subset "only" means that any other conditions being met must be excluded. Therefore, although *B* is composed of 2, 3, and 4, only 3 may be accepted, as 2 is also a subset of *A* and 4 is also a subset of *C*.

43. **The correct answer is (B).**

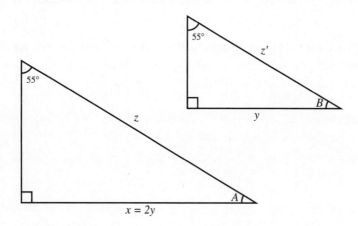

The ratio of the areas of similar triangles is equal to the square of the ratio of corresponding sides. Therefore, when $x = 2y$, the ratio of the sides is $\frac{2}{1} : \frac{x}{y}$ as *x* is twice the value of *y*. The ratio of the areas is then $\left(\frac{2}{1}\right)^2$ or $\frac{4}{1}$ or 4:1.

44. **The correct answer is (D).**

    The sum of all angles in a triangle is 180°. If one angle is 55° and a right angle is 90°, then angle *A* is 180° – 55° – 90° = 35°.

45. **The correct answer is (D).**

    Since the two triangles are similar, if $x = 3y$, then

    $z = 3\,z'$, or

    $$z' = \frac{z}{3} = \frac{5}{3} = 1\frac{2}{3}$$

46. **The correct answer is (B).**

The value of a bar graph is determined by drawing a line perpendicular to the y axis from the top of the graph. The point of interception is the y-value of that bar.

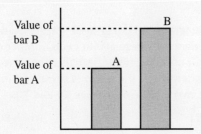

Therefore, only B and C have 90% or more of the active ingredient as declared by the manufacturer.

47. **The correct answer is (C).**

If sample B was 100% of claim and C was 120%, then the amount of drug present is

$$100\% \times 200 \text{ mg.} = 1 \times 200 = 200 \text{ mg.}$$

$$120\% \times 200 \text{ mg.} = 1.2 \times 200 = 240 \text{ mg.}$$

48. **The correct answer is (C).**

The mean is the sum of all values divided by the number of samples:

$\overline{X} = \dfrac{1}{N} \Sigma\, x$ when N is the number of samples and x is the value of each sample. From the bar graph, the following values were obtained:

1 score of 20	20 = (1 × 20)	5 scores of 70	350 = (5 × 70)
1 score of 30	30 = (1 × 30)	4 scores of 80	320 = (4 × 80)
1 score of 40	40 = (1 × 40)	2 scores of 90	180 = (2 × 90)
2 scores of 50	100 = (2 × 50)	1 score of 100	100 = (1 × 100)
3 scores of 60	180 = (3 × 60)		

$N = 20$ = number of samples Σ of all values = 1,320

$$\frac{1}{N} \Sigma\, x = \frac{1,320}{20} = 66 = \text{mean}$$

49.   The correct answer is (A).

The *modal score* is the most frequently occurring score. As 5 students scored 70% and no other score occurred as frequently, 70% is the modal score.

50.   The correct answer is (A).

The *median* is the term that is larger than or equal to half the terms and equal to or smaller than the other half of them. In this example, there are scores for a total of 20 students. As there are an even number of terms, there exists no actual median; that is, no term larger than exactly half of the terms and smaller than the other half. But now it is possible to find two middle terms, and the median is defined as the mean of these two middle terms. In this example, if the scores are ranked in ascending order, the two middle scores are 70 and 70:

1.	20	6.	60	*11.	70	16.	80
2.	30	7.	60	12.	70	17.	80
3.	40	8.	60	13.	70	18.	90
4.	50	9.	70	14.	80	19.	90
5.	50	*10.	70	15.	80	20.	100

*As rank position, 10 and 11 are in the middle; that is, 70 is larger than or equal to half of the terms and equal to or smaller than half, and as 70 is the mean of 70 and 70, the median is 70.

51.   The correct answer is (A).

This is a proportionality problem:

$$0.625 \text{ g.} : 50 :: 31.25 \text{ g.} : x$$

$$\frac{0.625}{50} = \frac{31.25}{x}$$

$$x \text{ tablets} = \frac{31.25 \text{ g.} \times 50 \text{ tablets}}{0.625 \text{ g.}}$$

$$= 2,500 \text{ tablets}$$

52.   The correct answer is (B).

Assuming that the dose should be directly related to body weight, we set up a proportion:

$$\frac{70 \text{ μg.}}{150 \text{ lbs.}} = \frac{x \text{ μg.}}{44 \text{ lbs.}}$$

$$x \text{ μg} = \frac{70 \text{ μg.} \times 44 \text{ lbs.}}{150 \text{ lbs.}}$$

$$x = 20.53 \text{ μg.} \cong 20 \text{ μg.}$$

53. The correct answer is (B).

To solve for changes in y relative to x, rearrange the equation in terms of y:

$$x = \frac{1}{y}$$

$$y = \frac{1}{x}$$

Then, substitute in the change:

$$y = \frac{1}{x(2)} = \left(\frac{1}{x}\right) \times \frac{1}{2}$$

Therefore, it can be seen that when x increases by a factor of 2, y is halved.

54. The correct answer is (A).

Rearrange the equation in terms of y (see above):

$$x = 2y$$

$$y = \frac{x}{2}$$

Increase x by a factor of 2:

$$y = \frac{x \times 2}{2}$$

y has increased by a factor of 2.

55. The correct answer is (D).

This is a simple fraction problem. The question is, how many times does 16 go into 24?

$$\frac{24 \text{ g.}}{16} = 1.5 \text{ g.} = 1{,}500 \text{ mg.}$$

56. The correct answer is (D).

Determine the weight that represents a 10% error. The range of acceptable weights would be all the tablet weights that are within 150 g. ± the 10% error:

$$150 \text{ g.} \times \frac{10\%}{100\%} = 15 \text{ g.}$$

$$150 \text{ g.} - 15 \text{ g.} = 135 \text{ g.}$$

$$150 \text{ g.} + 15 \text{ g.} = 165 \text{ g.}$$

So, the range is 135–165 g.

57. The correct answer is (A).

A percentage is the amount per hundred. A proportion should then be set up to find how much iron is in 100 mg. of ferrous sulfate, knowing the ratio of 65 mg./325 mg., iron to ferrous sulfate:

$$\frac{x}{100\%} = \frac{65 \text{ mg. of iron}}{325 \text{ mg. of ferrous sulfate}}$$

$$\frac{65 \text{ mg.}}{325 \text{ mg.}} \times 100\% = 20\%$$

58. The correct answer is (D).

Set up a proportion with x representing the number of milligrams of compound in a liter (remember, 1 liter equals 1,000 ml.):

$$\frac{x \text{ mg.}}{1,000 \text{ ml.}} = \frac{50 \text{ mg.}}{\text{ml.}}$$

$$x \text{ mg.} = \frac{50 \text{ mg.} \times 1,000 \text{ ml.}}{\text{ml.}}$$

$$= 50,000 \text{ mg.}$$

As 1,000 mg. are in 1 g.,

$$\frac{50,000 \text{ g.}}{1,000 \text{ mg.}/1 \text{ g.}} = 50 \text{ g.}$$

59. The correct answer is (B).

If 5 ml. is the smallest unit marked, then all errors are related to this unit and all readings would be rounded off to multiples of that unit; 5 ml. represents the potential error. In this problem, the potential error is also the percentage error of a measured volume (x ml.):

$$\frac{5 \text{ ml.}}{x \text{ ml.}} \times 100\% = \text{percentage error}$$

$$\frac{500\%}{x \text{ ml.}} = 10\%$$

$$x \text{ ml.} = \frac{500\%}{10\%}$$

$$x = 50 \text{ ml.}$$

60. The correct answer is (B).

The average is analogous to the mean:

$$\frac{1}{N} \Sigma \text{ values} = \text{average}$$

$$\frac{61 + 50 + 100 + 50}{1 + 1 + 1 + 1} = 65.25 = 65$$

88

61. **The correct answer is (C).**

The equation for a straight line is $y = mx + b$, where b is the y intercept and m is the slope. Thus,

$$y = mx + b$$

$$y = -0.118x + 8.5$$

62. **The correct answer is (A).**

Rearrange the equation of the line to isolate x; then, substitute the value of the y-intercept:

$$y = -0.118x + 8.5$$

$$y - 8.5 = -0.118x$$

$$\left[\frac{y - 8.5}{-0.118}\right] = x$$

$$\left[\frac{6 - 8.5}{-0.118}\right] = x$$

$$21 = x$$

63. **The correct answer is (C).**

The value of y, when x is zero, is 8.5. For all other values of x, solve for y by substituting into the equation of the line.

64. **The correct answer is (C).**

The volume of the cylinder is $\pi r^2 h$, where h (height) is 10 and r (radius) is 2:

$$\text{volume} = \pi r^2 h$$

$$= (3.14)(2^2)(10)$$

$$= 125.6 \text{ units}^3$$

$$= 126 \text{ units}^3$$

65. **The correct answer is (C).**

The lateral surface area is the circumference of the end, $2\pi r$, times the height:

$$\text{Lateral surface} = (2\pi r)(h)$$

$$= (2)(3.14)(2)(10)$$

$$= 125.6$$

$$= 126 \text{ units}^2$$

66. The correct answer is (B).

The total area is the area of the lateral surface plus the areas of both ends:

area of circle = πr^2

lateral surface = $2\pi rh$

total area = $(2)(\pi r^2) + (2\pi rh)$

$= 2\pi r \,(r + h)$

$= (2)\,(3.14)\,(2)\,(2 + 10)$

$= 150.7$

$= 151$ units^2

67. The correct answer is (B).

The area of a trapezoid is $\frac{1}{2}(h)\,(a + b)$:

$\frac{1}{2}(1)\,(4 + 2) = $ area

3 units$^2 = $ area

68. The correct answer is (C).

The area of a parallelogram is determined by $h \times b$:

$(2)(5) = $ area

10 units$^2 = $ area

69. The correct answer is (C).

To solve simultaneous equations, isolate the term in the first equation, which will be subsequently inserted into the second equation. In this case, y will be expressed in terms of x and b. The a term is common to both; therefore, rearrange the x equation to isolate a:

$x = 3b + a$

$a = x - 3b$

Then, substitute into the y equation:

$y = 3a + b = 3(x - 3b) + b$

$= 3x - 9b + b = 3x - 8b$

70. The correct answer is (A).

The slope of a line (m) is the change in y versus the change in x (x versus y). The ordinate (y-value) intercept is given by c. The abscissa (x-value) intercept occurs when y equals zero or $0 = mx + c$, $x = \frac{-c}{m}$.

71.   The correct answer is (D).

When one divides ratios with the same denominator, the denominators may be factored out and only the numerators divided. It may be viewed in any of the following fashions:

$$\frac{7 \div 3}{21 \div 3} = \frac{7}{21} = \frac{1}{3} = 0.33$$

$$7 : 3 :: 21 : 3 \rightarrow \frac{7}{21} = \frac{1}{3} = 0.33$$

$$\frac{7}{3} \div \frac{21}{3} = \frac{7}{21} = \frac{1}{3} = 0.33$$

72.   The correct answer is (D).

To reduce a fraction, first determine what roots of the numerator are common in the denominator:

$$\frac{72}{2,880} = \frac{72}{72 \times 40} \text{ or } \frac{2 \times 2 \times 2 \times 3 \times 3}{2 \times 2 \times 2 \times 2 \times 2 \times 2 \times 3 \times 3 \times 5}$$

$$= \frac{1}{2 \times 2 \times 2 \times 5}$$

$$= \frac{1}{40}$$

73.   The correct answer is (A).

Set up the proportion:

$$\frac{0.25 \text{ mg.}}{\text{tablet}} = \frac{7.5 \text{ mg.}}{x \text{ tablets}}$$

$$x = \frac{7.5 \text{ mg.} \times 1 \text{ tablet}}{0.25 \text{ mg.}}$$

$$x = 30$$

74.   The correct answer is (C).

Convert all the fractions to decimals; then, add all values:

$$\frac{3}{4} = \frac{x}{1.00} \qquad \frac{2}{5} = \frac{x}{1.00}$$

$$x = \frac{3 \times 1.00}{4} \qquad x = \frac{2 \times 1.00}{5}$$

$$x = 0.75 \qquad x = 0.40$$

$$\frac{3}{4} \text{ mg.} + 0.25 \text{ mg.} + \frac{2}{5} \text{ mg.} + 2.75 \text{ mg.} = x \text{ mg.}$$

$$0.75 + 0.25 + 0.40 + 2.75 = 4.15 \text{ mg.}$$

75.   The correct answer is (A).

To add, convert all numbers to common units. In this case, grams (g.) is the base unit:

$$1,000 \text{ mg.} = 1 \text{ g.}$$

$$1 \text{ kg.} = 1,000 \text{ g.}$$

Therefore,

$$\frac{0.75 \text{ mg.}}{x \text{ g.}} = \frac{1,000 \text{ mg.}}{1 \text{ g.}}$$

$$x \text{ g.} = 0.00075 \text{ g.}$$

$$\frac{0.5 \text{ kg.}}{x \text{ g.}} = \frac{1 \text{ kg.}}{1,000 \text{ g.}}$$

$$x \text{ g.} = 500 \text{ g.}$$

$$0.75 \text{ mg.} + 50 \text{ g.} + 0.5 \text{ kg.} - x \text{ g.}$$

$$0.00075 \text{ g.} + 50 \text{ g.} + 500 \text{ g.} = 550.00075 \text{ g.}$$

76.   The correct answer is (B).

Express $3\frac{1}{8}$ as a fraction:

$$\frac{3 \times 8}{8} + \frac{1}{8} = \frac{25}{8}$$

Then, convert the fraction so that it has a denominator common to those of the possible answers. Those values with a denominator of 36 may automatically be discarded, as 8 is not a factor of 36, (i.e., 36 cannot be divided by 8 to yield a whole number). Therefore, only denominators of 32 need be considered:

$$\frac{25 \times 4}{8 \times 4} = \frac{100}{32}$$

77.   The correct answer is (B).

First determine how many milligrams are being considered; then convert to grains by proportionalities:

$$\frac{10\%}{100\%} \times 360 = 36 \text{ mg.}$$

$$\frac{1 \text{ g.}}{60 \text{ mg.}} = \frac{x \text{ g.}}{36 \text{ mg.}}$$

$$x \text{ grains} = 0.6 \text{ grain}$$

78. The correct answer is (D).

Both quantities must first be converted to similar denominators; then, they can be simplified and added:

$$\frac{2\sqrt{36}\times 3\sqrt{7}}{3\sqrt{7}}+\frac{4\sqrt{28}}{3\sqrt{7}}=\frac{\left(2\sqrt{6\times 6}\times 3\sqrt{7}\right)}{3\sqrt{7}}+\frac{4\sqrt{2\times 2\times 7}}{3\sqrt{7}}$$

$$=\frac{(2\times 6)\times\left(3\sqrt{7}\right)+4\sqrt{2\times 2}\times\sqrt{7}}{3\sqrt{7}}$$

$$=\frac{36+8}{3}$$

$$=14\frac{2}{3}$$

79. The correct answer is (A).

This is a simple subtraction problem. If A were equal to x, then $1 + A$ would equal $1 + x$. The value of A does not change the mathematical principle. Therefore, when

$$A = e^a$$

we have

$$1 + A = 1 + e^a$$

80. The correct answer is (C).

Any number to the power of zero is 1:

$$7.7 \times 10^0 = 7.7 \times 1 = 7.7$$

81. The correct answer is (C).

1,000,000 expressed in base 10 is 1×10^6. Using the law of exponents (see Answer 19), we have

$$1 \times 10^3 \times 10^3 = 1 \times 10^{3+3}$$

$$= 1 \times 10^6$$

82. The correct answer is (D).

Using the law of exponents (see Answer 19), we see that $\sqrt{144\times 10^4}$ may be broken down as follows:

$$\sqrt{144\times 10^4}=\sqrt{144}\times\sqrt{10^4}$$

$$=\sqrt{12\times 12}\times\sqrt{10^2\times 10^2}$$

$$=12\times 10^2$$

$$=1,200$$

83. The correct answer is (A).

Using proportionalities to convert the total weight after summing, we have 132 lbs. + 11 lbs. + 44 lbs. = 187 lbs. So, then

$$\frac{1 \text{ kg.}}{2.2 \text{ lbs.}} = \frac{x \text{ kg.}}{187 \text{ lbs.}}$$

$$\frac{1 \text{ kg.} \times 187 \text{ lbs.}}{2.2 \text{ lbs.}} = x \text{ kg.}$$

$$x \text{ kg.} = 85 \text{ kg.}$$

84. The correct answer is (B).

Simply convert to a common denominator and add (see Answer 19):

$$\left(\frac{3}{4}\right)^2 = \frac{3^2}{4^2} = \frac{9}{16}$$

$$3^2 = 9$$

$$\sqrt{\frac{49}{256}} = \frac{\sqrt{49}}{\sqrt{256}} = \frac{\sqrt{7 \times 7}}{\sqrt{2 \times 2 \times 2 \times 2 \times 2 \times 2 \times 2 \times 2}}$$

$$= \frac{7}{\sqrt{2^8}} = \frac{7}{\sqrt{2^4}} = \frac{7}{16}$$

Therefore,

$$\frac{3^2}{4} + 3^2 + \sqrt{\frac{49}{256}} = x$$

$$\frac{9}{16} + \frac{9 \times 16}{16} + \frac{7}{16} = x$$

$$x = \frac{160}{16} = 10$$

85. The correct answer is (C).

The equation of a line is $y = mx + b$ (see Answers 26–28), where m is the slope and b is the y-intercept. Therefore,

$$y = mx + b$$

$$y = -2x + \sqrt{2}$$

86. The correct answer is (D).

Simplify the numerator; then, divide the result by the denominator:

$$250,000 \times 0.018 = 4,500.000. = 4,500$$

$$\frac{4,500}{0.15} = 30,000.00$$

$$= 30,000$$

87. The correct answer is (A).

If we use the law of exponents, $x^{-3} = \dfrac{1}{x^3}$, then

$$\frac{1}{x^3} = \frac{1}{27}$$
$$x^3 = 27$$
$$x = \sqrt[3]{27} = \sqrt[3]{3 \times 3 \times 3}$$
$$= 3$$

88. The correct answer is (A).

Corresponding sides of similar triangles are related by the same ratio. Therefore,

$$\frac{J}{K} = \text{ratio of one side}$$

$$\frac{H}{I} = \text{ratio of second side}$$

$$\frac{J}{K} = \frac{H}{I}$$

$$I = \frac{KH}{J}$$

89. The correct answer is (A).

If drug A is 20% of the compound, then drug A is 20% of 500 g.

$$\frac{20\%}{100\%} \times 500 = \text{grams of drug A}$$

$$\frac{10,000}{100} = \text{grams of drug A} = 100$$

90. The correct answer is (B).

Drugs A and B represent 20% and 5%, respectively, of the compound. Therefore, 25% of 500 g. is the amount of drugs A and B.

$$\frac{20}{100} + \frac{5}{100} \times 500 \text{ g.} = \text{grams of drugs A and B}$$

$$\frac{12,500}{100} = \text{grams of drugs A and B} = 125 \text{ g.}$$

91. The correct answer is (D).

Drugs B and C represent 5% and 75% of the compound. Therefore, 80% of 500 g. is the amount of drugs B and C.

$$\frac{5}{100} + \frac{75}{100} \times 500 \text{ g.} = \text{grams of drugs B and C}$$

$$\frac{40,000}{100} = \text{grams of drugs B and C} = 400$$

92. The correct answer is (A).

Drugs A, B, and C represent 20%, 5%, and 75% of the compound, which, when summed, make up 100% of the compound. Therefore, 100 g. of drugs A, B, and C are in 100 g. of the compound.

93. The correct answer is (B).

The ratios A:B:C are 20%:5%:75%.

If 5 is the lowest common denominator, then

$$\frac{20}{5} : \frac{5}{5} : \frac{75}{5}$$

or, 4:1:15

94. The correct answer is (D).

If this problem is approached as a proportion, then the product of the means divided by one of the extremes equals the other extreme. Initially, isolate the extreme $g_b M_b$:

$$\frac{B-p}{q} = \frac{g_b M_a}{g_b M_b}$$

$$g_b M_b = \frac{(g_a M_a)(q)}{B-p}$$

Again, treat the equation as a proportion and isolate the extreme (g_b):

$$g_b = \frac{(g_a M_a)(q)(M_b)}{B-p}$$

that upon rearrangement, yields

$$g_b = \left[\frac{q}{B-p}\right]\left[\frac{M_b(g_a)}{M_a}\right]$$

95.   The correct answer is (D).

From the equation for a straight line (see Answers 26–28), $y = mx + b$:

	y-intercept (b)	slope (m)	x-intercept ($y = 0$)
Equation 1	4	+3	$-\dfrac{4}{3}$
Equation 2	–4	+3	$\dfrac{4}{3}$

96.   The correct answer is (A).

To solve simultaneous equations, express the first equation in terms of a single unknown term (I). Then, substitute this value into the second equation and solve for the second unknown (II). After solving for the second unknown, substitute its value back into the first equation and solve for the remaining unknown term (III):

(I)

$$30 = a + 3b - 70$$

$$a = 30 - 3b + 70$$

(II)

$$3a + 5b = 100$$

$$3(30 - 3b + 70) + 5b = 100$$

$$90 - 9b + 210 + 5b = 100$$

$$-4b = 100 - 210 - 90$$

$$4b = 200$$

$$b = 50$$

(III)

$$30 = a + 3b - 70$$

$$30 = a + 3(50) - 70$$

$$30 = a + 150 - 70$$

$$a = -50$$

97.   The correct answer is (B).

The question is really asking what is the total volume used. This is the total volume of a dose times the number of doses, which is then expressed in milliliters:

$$\frac{2 \text{ tablespoonfuls}}{\text{dose}} \times \frac{2 \text{ doses}}{\text{day}} \times 10 \text{ days} = \text{total volume}$$

$$40 \text{ tablespoonfuls} \times \frac{15 \text{ ml.}}{\text{tablespoonful}} = 600 \text{ ml.}$$

98. The correct answer is (D).

This problem is solved with proportions; however, as we will be dividing the total weight into smaller units, the weight should be converted to a smaller unit to minimize the number of decimal places of which we will have to keep track:

$$0.060 \text{ g.} \times \frac{1,000 \text{ mg.}}{1 \text{ g.}} = 60 \text{ mg.}$$

$$\frac{60 \text{ mg.}}{125 \text{ tablets}} = \frac{x \text{ mg.}}{\text{tablet}}$$

$$0.480 \text{ mg.} = \frac{x \text{ mg.}}{\text{tablet}}$$

$$0.480 \text{ mg.} \times \frac{1,000 \text{ g.}}{\text{mg.}} = 480 \text{ g.}$$

99. The correct answer is (C).

This is a conversion problem, which again, is easiest to solve by the use of proportions:

$$\frac{1 \text{ in.}}{2.54 \text{ cm.}} = \frac{x \text{ in.}}{12.70 \text{ cm.}}$$

$$\frac{12.70 \times 1 \text{ in.}}{2.54 \text{ cm.}} = x \text{ in.}$$

$$5 \text{ in.} = x$$

100. The correct answer is (A).

To divide fractions, invert the second term and multiply:

$$\frac{1}{120} \div \frac{1}{150} = \frac{1}{120} \times \frac{150}{1} = \frac{150}{120}$$

Then, simplify and complete the multiplication:

$$\frac{150}{120} = \frac{15}{12} = \frac{5 \times 3}{4 \times 3} = \frac{5}{4}$$

$$\frac{5}{4} \times 50 = \frac{250}{4} = 62\frac{1}{2}$$

Chapter 8: Biology

KEY POINTS TO REMEMBER

The ultimate goal of pharmaceutical care is to optimize therapeutic outcomes, i.e., reduce the incidence of adverse side effects while at the same time increasing drug efficiency via individualization of drug therapy. To this end, a pharmacist must understand how drugs act on the body (pharmacology), how the body acts on drugs (pharmacokinetics), and how disease (pathophysiology) affects a drug's pharmacology and pharmacokinetics.

To be prepared for the academic rigors of pharmacy school, you must have a good background in the disciplines of cellular and molecular biology, anatomy and physiology, and biochemistry. In fact, studies have shown that a student's performance on the Biology Section of the PCAT is a good predictor of academic success in pharmacy school. Below is a breakdown of the major points you will need to know for the Biology Section of the PCAT:

1) **Molecular Cell Biology**

   a) All animal cells are comprised of a cell membrane, cytoplasm, cytoplasmic organelles, and a nucleus.

   b) Fluid Mosaic Model

   c) Integral proteins are intimately associated with the membrane lipids and cannot be extracted from the membrane without membrane disruption.

   d) Membrane proteins are located on the cytoplasmic surface of the cell and are associated with cell shape and motility.

   e) Cytoplasmic organelles

   f) Membrane Transport

   g) Cell Cycle

   h) Cellular Respiration

   i) Molecular Biology

2) **Organ Systems**

   a) Tissue organization

       i) The four major types of tissue include epithelial, connective, muscle, and nervous.

       ii) Extracellular fluid is comprised of interstitial fluid and plasma.

       iii) The three types of cell junctions include tight junctions, desmosomes, and gap junctions.

       iv) Exocrine glandular secretions

b) Skeletal system

    i) Function: support, protection of underlying organs, movement, mineral and energy storage, and hematopoiesis

    ii) Organs: bones, tendons, ligaments, and cartilage

c) Muscular system

    i) Function: locomotion and manipulation, vision, facial expression (skeletal), blood pumping (cardiac), food digesting, urination (smooth), posture, joint stability, and heat generation

    ii) Organs: skeletal muscles

    iii) Smooth Muscle System

d) Cardiovascular system

    i) Function: transport nutrients and O_2 to tissues and remove cellular wastes (e.g., urea and CO_2)

    ii) Organs: heart and blood vessels

e) Respiratory system

    i) Function: exchange of gases (O_2 and CO_2); maintenance of blood pH and electrolytes

    ii) Organs: oral cavity, nose, nasal cavity, pharynx, larynx, trachea, bronchial tubes within lungs, and alveoli

f) Urinary system

    i) Function: removal of metabolic wastes from blood, maintenance of blood, pH, and electrolytes

    ii) Organs: kidneys, ureters, urinary bladder, and urethra

g) Integumentary system

    i) Function: protection, excretion, regulation of body temperature, sensory reception, immunity, synthesis of Vitamin D, and blood reservoir

    ii) Organs: skin, hair, nails, sweat glands, and sebaceous glands

h) Digestive system

    i) Function: breakdown of food into substances that can be absorbed for energy

    ii) Organs: mouth, pharynx, esophagus, stomach, small and large intestine, salivary glands, liver, pancreas, and gall bladder

i) Nervous system

    i) Function: The general function of the nervous system is to coordinate all body systems. This is accomplished by the transmission of (electrochemical) signals from body parts to the brain and back to the body parts; coordination of body parts; control

    ii) Organs: brain, spinal cord, and nerves

j) Endocrine system

    i) Function: to integrate body systems (i.e. maintain homeostasis) in conjunction with the nervous system

    ii) Organs: endocrine glands (hypothalamus, pituitary, pineal gland, thyroid, parathyroids, thymus, adrenals, pancreas, testes, and ovaries) that secrete hormones

k) Reproductive system

    i) Function: production, maintenance, and transport of gametes; production of sex hormones

    ii) Organs: male: testes, epididymis, vas deferens, prostate, seminal vesicle, bulbourethral glands, urethra, penis, and scrotum. Female: ovaries, fallopian tubes, uterus, cervix, vagina, labia, and clitoris

l) Lymphatic system

    i) Function: to prevent edema (accumulation of excess tissue fluid), transport dietary fat, and help fight infection

    ii) Organs: primary (bone marrow and thymus); secondary (lymph nodes and spleen)

m) Somatic sensory system

    i) Function: process sensation and perception

Answer Sheet

Chapter 8: Biology

Tear Here

1. Ⓐ Ⓑ Ⓒ Ⓓ   16. Ⓐ Ⓑ Ⓒ Ⓓ   31. Ⓐ Ⓑ Ⓒ Ⓓ   46. Ⓐ Ⓑ Ⓒ Ⓓ   61. Ⓐ Ⓑ Ⓒ Ⓓ

2. Ⓐ Ⓑ Ⓒ Ⓓ   17. Ⓐ Ⓑ Ⓒ Ⓓ   32. Ⓐ Ⓑ Ⓒ Ⓓ   47. Ⓐ Ⓑ Ⓒ Ⓓ   62. Ⓐ Ⓑ Ⓒ Ⓓ

3. Ⓐ Ⓑ Ⓒ Ⓓ   18. Ⓐ Ⓑ Ⓒ Ⓓ   33. Ⓐ Ⓑ Ⓒ Ⓓ   48. Ⓐ Ⓑ Ⓒ Ⓓ   63. Ⓐ Ⓑ Ⓒ Ⓓ

4. Ⓐ Ⓑ Ⓒ Ⓓ   19. Ⓐ Ⓑ Ⓒ Ⓓ   34. Ⓐ Ⓑ Ⓒ Ⓓ   49. Ⓐ Ⓑ Ⓒ Ⓓ   64. Ⓐ Ⓑ Ⓒ Ⓓ

5. Ⓐ Ⓑ Ⓒ Ⓓ   20. Ⓐ Ⓑ Ⓒ Ⓓ   35. Ⓐ Ⓑ Ⓒ Ⓓ   50. Ⓐ Ⓑ Ⓒ Ⓓ   65. Ⓐ Ⓑ Ⓒ Ⓓ

6. Ⓐ Ⓑ Ⓒ Ⓓ   21. Ⓐ Ⓑ Ⓒ Ⓓ   36. Ⓐ Ⓑ Ⓒ Ⓓ   51. Ⓐ Ⓑ Ⓒ Ⓓ   66. Ⓐ Ⓑ Ⓒ Ⓓ

7. Ⓐ Ⓑ Ⓒ Ⓓ   22. Ⓐ Ⓑ Ⓒ Ⓓ   37. Ⓐ Ⓑ Ⓒ Ⓓ   52. Ⓐ Ⓑ Ⓒ Ⓓ   67. Ⓐ Ⓑ Ⓒ Ⓓ

8. Ⓐ Ⓑ Ⓒ Ⓓ   23. Ⓐ Ⓑ Ⓒ Ⓓ   38. Ⓐ Ⓑ Ⓒ Ⓓ   53. Ⓐ Ⓑ Ⓒ Ⓓ   68. Ⓐ Ⓑ Ⓒ Ⓓ

9. Ⓐ Ⓑ Ⓒ Ⓓ   24. Ⓐ Ⓑ Ⓒ Ⓓ   39. Ⓐ Ⓑ Ⓒ Ⓓ   54. Ⓐ Ⓑ Ⓒ Ⓓ   69. Ⓐ Ⓑ Ⓒ Ⓓ

10. Ⓐ Ⓑ Ⓒ Ⓓ   25. Ⓐ Ⓑ Ⓒ Ⓓ   40. Ⓐ Ⓑ Ⓒ Ⓓ   55. Ⓐ Ⓑ Ⓒ Ⓓ   70. Ⓐ Ⓑ Ⓒ Ⓓ

11. Ⓐ Ⓑ Ⓒ Ⓓ   26. Ⓐ Ⓑ Ⓒ Ⓓ   41. Ⓐ Ⓑ Ⓒ Ⓓ   56. Ⓐ Ⓑ Ⓒ Ⓓ   71. Ⓐ Ⓑ Ⓒ Ⓓ

12. Ⓐ Ⓑ Ⓒ Ⓓ   27. Ⓐ Ⓑ Ⓒ Ⓓ   42. Ⓐ Ⓑ Ⓒ Ⓓ   57. Ⓐ Ⓑ Ⓒ Ⓓ   72. Ⓐ Ⓑ Ⓒ Ⓓ

13. Ⓐ Ⓑ Ⓒ Ⓓ   28. Ⓐ Ⓑ Ⓒ Ⓓ   43. Ⓐ Ⓑ Ⓒ Ⓓ   58. Ⓐ Ⓑ Ⓒ Ⓓ   73. Ⓐ Ⓑ Ⓒ Ⓓ

14. Ⓐ Ⓑ Ⓒ Ⓓ   29. Ⓐ Ⓑ Ⓒ Ⓓ   44. Ⓐ Ⓑ Ⓒ Ⓓ   59. Ⓐ Ⓑ Ⓒ Ⓓ   74. Ⓐ Ⓑ Ⓒ Ⓓ

15. Ⓐ Ⓑ Ⓒ Ⓓ   30. Ⓐ Ⓑ Ⓒ Ⓓ   45. Ⓐ Ⓑ Ⓒ Ⓓ   60. Ⓐ Ⓑ Ⓒ Ⓓ   75. Ⓐ Ⓑ Ⓒ Ⓓ

Biology Practice Questions

75 QUESTIONS—45 MINUTES
Directions: Choose the best answer to each of the following questions.

1. The smallest unit of life is the
   (A) organ.
   (B) organelle.
   (C) cell.
   (D) gene.

2. The organelle primarily responsible for energy production in an aerobic cell is the
   (A) nucleus.
   (B) mitochondria.
   (C) endoplasmic reticulum.
   (D) Golgi apparatus.

3. In humans, brown eyes (*B*) are dominant over blue eyes (*b*). In a cross between two *Bb* individuals, what percentage of offspring will have blue eyes?
   (A) 0 percent
   (B) 25 percent
   (C) 75 percent
   (D) 100 percent

4. Solutions that cause red blood cells to shrink are called
   (A) isotonic.
   (B) iso-osmotic.
   (C) hypertonic.
   (D) hypotonic.

5. A trace element necessary for normal health of the human body is
   (A) sodium.
   (B) potassium.
   (C) calcium.
   (D) copper.

6. Brown is the dominant color for rats, whereas white is the alternative recessive color. When a homozygous brown rat is crossed with a homozygous white rat, what percentage of the offspring is expected to be brown heterozygous?
   (A) 25 percent
   (B) 50 percent
   (C) 75 percent
   (D) 100 percent

7. Fat-soluble vitamins include all of the following EXCEPT Vitamin
   (A) A
   (B) B
   (C) D
   (D) K

8. Under basal conditions, the region of the body that receives the greatest blood flow is the
   (A) liver.
   (B) brain.
   (C) bone.
   (D) skeletal muscle.

9. Which of the following electrolytes is most abundant in human extracellular fluid?
   (A) Sodium
   (B) Potassium
   (C) Calcium
   (D) Magnesium

10. Most nutrients are absorbed by which region of the human gastrointestinal tract?
    (A) Stomach
    (B) Colon
    (C) Small intestine
    (D) Large intestine

11. Long-chain fatty acids normally enter the blood system in the form of
    (A) cholesterol esters.
    (B) free fatty acids.
    (C) glycoproteins.
    (D) chylomicrons.

12. The most abundant electrolyte in the intracellular fluid of humans is
    (A) sodium.
    (B) potassium.
    (C) calcium.
    (D) magnesium.

13. In humans, a deficiency in Vitamin C (ascorbic acid) is normally associated with
    (A) scurvy.
    (B) rickets.
    (C) pellagra.
    (D) beriberi.

14. Squamous epithelium is normally associated with which region of the human body?
    (A) Kidney
    (B) Lungs
    (C) Skin
    (D) Pancreas

15. Which of the following statements concerning the structure of a cell is false?
    (A) The nucleus of a cell contains DNA and is separated from the surrounding cytoplasm by a nuclear membrane.
    (B) The Golgi apparatus, endoplasmic reticulum, and the majority of chromatin are found in the cytoplasm outside the nucleus.
    (C) A cell with two complete sets of chromosomes is diploid.
    (D) None of the above

16. Which type of muscle will contract most rapidly when stimulated?
    (A) Skeletal
    (B) Cardiac
    (C) Smooth
    (D) All muscle types contract at the same rate.

17. Which statement about fatty acids (triglycerides) is true?

    (A) Most fats containing unsaturated fatty acids are solids at room temperature, whereas fats containing saturated fatty acids are liquids.

    (B) Most fatty acids in nature have an even number of carbon atoms.

    (C) Fats yield approximately 50% as much energy as do carbohydrates in humans.

    (D) Saturated fatty acids contain one or more double carbon bonds.

18. The nucleic acid responsible for transmitting genetic information from the DNA molecule in the nucleus to the cytoplasm is

    (A) transfer RNA.

    (B) ribosomal RNA.

    (C) messenger RNA.

    (D) None of the above

19. The proper sequence for the stages of mitosis is

    (A) metaphase, prophase, anaphase, and telophase.

    (B) prophase, anaphase, metaphase, and telophase.

    (C) prophase, metaphase, telophase, and anaphase.

    (D) prophase, metaphase, anaphase, and telophase.

20. Which statement concerning the structure and function of the biological membrane is true?

    (A) Biological membranes are primarily composed of protein with a small layer of lipid on both the inner and outer surfaces.

    (B) Lipid-soluble compounds tend to diffuse through biological membranes faster than water-soluble ones.

    (C) The rate at which lipid-soluble substances pass through biological membranes is determined by the size of the diffusing particle.

    (D) All of the above

21. Passive diffusion of substances through biological membranes

    (A) requires energy sources such as ATP.

    (B) causes a substance to move from a lower to a higher concentration.

    (C) can be inhibited by metabolic poisons such as cyanide.

    (D) is a major process by which uncharged molecules can move through membranes.

22. The ascending (initial) portion of an action potential observed in a cell is caused by

    (A) sodium influx into the cell.

    (B) sodium efflux out of the cell.

    (C) potassium influx into the cell.

    (D) potassium efflux out of the cell.

23. The descending portion of an action potential after the initial spike potential in a cell is caused by

    (A) sodium influx into the cell.

    (B) sodium efflux out of the cell.

    (C) potassium influx into the cell.

    (D) potassium efflux out of the cell.

24. The normal resting potential of the inner side of a nerve cell relative to the outer side is

    (A) 100 mV.

    (B) 50 mV.

    (C) –50 mV.

    (D) –500 mV.

25. Which of the following endogenous substances does NOT actively aid in the digestion of dietary nutrients?

    (A) Pepsin

    (B) Insulin

    (C) Lactase

    (D) Trypsin

26. The organ primarily responsible for detoxifying toxic substances in the blood is the

    (A) lung.

    (B) kidney.

    (C) liver.

    (D) pancreas.

27. In humans, the removal of waste products from the blood is one of the primary functions of the

    (A) liver.

    (B) pancreas.

    (C) kidneys.

    (D) spleen.

28. Absorption of dietary nutrients can be accomplished by which process?

    (A) Active transport

    (B) Facilitated diffusion

    (C) Passive diffusion

    (D) All of the above

29. In humans, bile salts play an important role in enhancing the intestinal absorption of

    (A) fatty acids.

    (B) glucose.

    (C) thiamine.

    (D) amino acids.

30. Which of the following sugars is NOT classified as a simple sugar that can be directly absorbed from the digestive tract in humans?

    (A) Glucose

    (B) Fructose

    (C) Glycogen

    (D) Galactose

31. Which organ of the human body is first affected by a rapid decrease of glucose concentration in the blood?

    (A) Brain

    (B) Heart

    (C) Kidneys

    (D) Eyes

32. In humans, night blindness can be due to a diet deficient in

    (A) iron.

    (B) copper.

    (C) Vitamin K.

    (D) Vitamin A.

33. The transport process that does not require the presence of a carrier is
    (A) active transport.
    (B) passive diffusion.
    (C) facilitated diffusion.
    (D) None of the above

34. Saturation kinetics are NOT usually observed in which of the following transport processes?
    (A) Active transport
    (B) Passive diffusion
    (C) Facilitated diffusion
    (D) Phagocytosis

35. Which theory states that genes exist in individuals as pairs?
    (A) The theory of recapitulation
    (B) Starling's law
    (C) Mendel's law of segregation
    (D) The Watson-Crick model

36. Of the following, the element least abundant in the human body is
    (A) carbon.
    (B) oxygen.
    (C) hydrogen.
    (D) calcium.

37. Each cell of every organism of a given species contains a characteristic number of chromosomes. How many chromosomes are found in each cell of the human body?
    (A) 13
    (B) 23
    (C) 46
    (D) 48

38. In humans, which blood type is known as the universal donor?
    (A) O negative
    (B) O positive
    (C) AB negative
    (D) AB positive

39. All of the following substances are known to be neurotransmitters at neuromuscular junctions EXCEPT
    (A) epinephrine.
    (B) norepinephrine.
    (C) acetylcholine.
    (D) cholecystokinin.

40. Certain white blood cells are produced in lymphoid tissue such as the spleen, thymus, and lymph nodes. Which of the following white blood cells is produced by lymphoid tissue?
    (A) Neutrophils
    (B) Monocytes
    (C) Eosinophils
    (D) None of the above

41. Immunity produced in response to vaccination with some foreign protein (antigen) is known as
    (A) actively acquired immunity.
    (B) passively acquired immunity.
    (C) natural immunity.
    (D) cellular immunity.

42. The major process by which the kidney removes waste products from the blood is called

(A) tubular secretion.

(B) tubular reabsorption.

(C) glomerular filtration.

(D) tubular sublimation.

43. Stimulation of the human sympathetic nervous system causes all of the following changes in the body EXCEPT

(A) increased heart rate.

(B) increased sweating.

(C) constriction of pupils.

(D) increased blood pressure.

44. Fatigue of a muscle that has contracted many times is primarily caused by an accumulation of

(A) carbon dioxide.

(B) lactic acid.

(C) urea.

(D) sodium chloride.

45. Cell division during which the chromosome number is reduced from diploid to haploid is known as

(A) mitosis.

(B) synapsis.

(C) meiosis.

(D) karyokinesis.

46. The appearance of any individual with respect to a given inherited trait is known as its

(A) genotype.

(B) phenotype.

(C) recessive trait.

(D) heterozygous trait.

47. Which of the following disease states is known to be caused by homozygous recessive genes in an individual?

(A) Sickle-cell anemia

(B) Beriberi

(C) Hypertension

(D) Pellagra

48. Intense exercise and training of an athlete can result in which of the following changes?

(A) Increase in the number of muscle fibers

(B) Increased respiratory rate

(C) Increase in the size of muscle fibers

(D) A and C

49. During sperm formation, spermatids

(A) develop directly from primary spermatocytes.

(B) contain the diploid number of chromosomes.

(C) develop immediately after the first meiotic division.

(D) develop immediately after the second meiotic division.

50. An individual with type A negative blood can receive blood from which of the following blood types?

(A) O negative

(B) A positive

(C) O positive

(D) All of the above

51. Vestigial organs are the remnants of organs that were functional in some ancestral animal. In humans, which organ(s) is NOT vestigial in nature?

   (A) Appendix

   (B) Wisdom teeth

   (C) Coccygeal vertebrae

   (D) Pupils of the eyes

52. Which of the following graphs most accurately shows the relation between the substrate (S) and product (P) in a saturated irreversible enzymatic reaction?

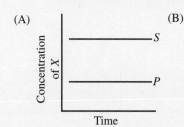 (A)

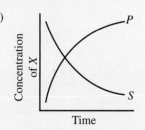 (B)

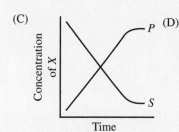 (C)

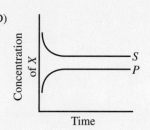 (D)

53. Oxygen and carbon dioxide are primarily transported through the blood

   (A) dissolved in plasma water.

   (B) bound to plasma proteins.

   (C) bound to hemoglobin.

   (D) None of the above

54. Which of the following statements is false concerning the genetics of humans and animals?

   (A) Inbreeding is harmful and leads to the production of genetically inferior offspring.

   (B) Defective traits can be sex linked.

   (C) Outbreeding is the mating of two totally unrelated individuals.

   (D) Vigorous inbreeding can result in a high frequency of defects present at birth, termed congenital anomalies.

55. The members of two different species of animals or plants that share the same living space or food source may interact with each other in a positive or negative manner. Which of the following would be a negative interaction?

   (A) Parasitism

   (B) Commensalism

   (C) Protocooperation

   (D) Mutualism

56. Which of the following graphs most accurately shows the relationship between the substrate (*S*) and product (*P*) in a reversible unsaturated enzymatic reaction?

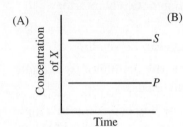 (A)

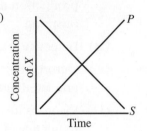 (B)

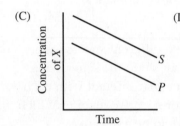 (C)

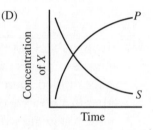 (D)

57. Which of the following plasma proteins is most responsible for the osmotic pressure that regulates the water content of the plasma?

(A) Fibrinogen

(B) Albumin

(C) Hemoglobin

(D) Gammaglobulin

58. Which of the following statements is false concerning leukocytes in the human body?

(A) Leukocytes are white blood cells.

(B) Leukocytes move actively by amoeboid movement.

(C) Leukocytes contain hemoglobin.

(D) There are the same number of leukocytes as erythrocytes in plasma.

59. Cells that are very important in the production of antibodies for the immune system are

(A) thrombocytes.

(B) megakaryocytes.

(C) neutrophils.

(D) plasma cells.

60. Which of the following graphs most accurately shows the relationship between the substrate (*S*) and product (*P*) in a saturated reversible enzymatic reaction after treatment with cyanide?

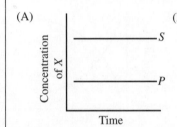 (A)

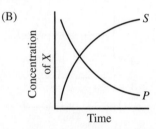 (B)

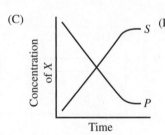 (C)

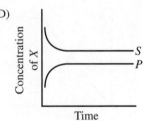 (D)

61. The transport of oxygen and carbon dioxide in the blood depends largely on which component of the red blood cell?

(A) Cell wall

(B) Nucleus

(C) Hemoglobin

(D) Cytoplasm

CHAPTER 8: BIOLOGY

62. The plasma protein most abundant in plasma is
   (A) albumin.
   (B) globulin.
   (C) fibrinogen.
   (D) immunoglobin.

63. Which of the following conditions does NOT increase the number of red blood cells in the human body?
   (A) High altitude environment
   (B) Low oxygen delivery to the tissues
   (C) Increased erythropoietin production
   (D) Increased carbon dioxide concentration in the blood

64. Which of the following is NOT associated with heat loss in humans?
   (A) Sweating
   (B) Increased muscle tone
   (C) Decreased metabolism
   (D) Vasodilation

65. Substances that are actively reabsorbed by the kidney tubules include
   (A) urea.
   (B) creatinine.
   (C) glucose.
   (D) All of the above

66. Tissues of the body that are normally involved in regulating the volume of body fluids do NOT include
   (A) baroreceptors.
   (B) vasomotor center of the brain.
   (C) osmoreceptor.
   (D) reticular activating system.

67. The structural and functional unit of the nervous system of all multicellular animals is the
   (A) axon.
   (B) nerve.
   (C) neuron.
   (D) dendrite.

68. Which of the following statements about the rate of conduction for a nerve impulse is true in humans?
   (A) The rate of conduction increases as the diameter of the axon increases.
   (B) The rate of conduction is faster in smaller nerve fibers than in larger ones.
   (C) Myelin sheaths usually decrease the rate of conduction.
   (D) All of the above

69. Which of the following statements concerning the human autonomic nervous system is true?
   (A) It controls the voluntary movements of muscles in the limbs.
   (B) It is composed of both sympathetic and parasympathetic nerves.
   (C) Motor impulses reach the effector organ from the brain or spinal cord by a single neuron.
   (D) All of the above

70. In humans, hormones that are derived from amino acids include
   (A) prostaglandins.
   (B) estradiol.
   (C) testosterone.
   (D) thyroxine.

71. When a skeletal muscle fiber is given a single stimulus, a single twitch with numerous electrical phases is observed. What is the correct order for the phases or periods seen in a skeletal muscle fiber after stimulation?

    (A) Contraction, latent, relaxation, refractory

    (B) Refractory, contraction, latent, relaxation

    (C) Latent, contraction, relaxation, refractory

    (D) Latent, refractory, contraction, relaxation

72. Which statement is false concerning the role of hormones in the human body?

    (A) Hormones can be secreted by one part of the body, pass through the blood, and act on a target organ in another part of the body.

    (B) Neurohormones may pass down axons to the target organ in another part of the body.

    (C) Hormones can be derivatives of amino acids, fatty acids, or long peptides.

    (D) Hormones usually provide instantaneous control of a bodily function.

73. Hormones for the regulation of the menstrual cycle in women include

    (A) progesterone.

    (B) vasopressin.

    (C) aldosterone.

    (D) None of the above

74. In the human eye, the rods located in the retina are responsible for

    (A) color vision.

    (B) bright light vision.

    (C) peripheral vision.

    (D) All of the above

75. Which of the following statements is NOT true in reference to the human lymphatic system?

    (A) The rate of lymph flow is similar to that of the circulation.

    (B) The lymphatic system is an auxiliary system for return of fluid from the tissue spaces to the circulation.

    (C) Lymph nodes produce one type of white blood cells, known as lymphocytes.

    (D) The lymphatic system plays an important role in the immune process.

ANSWER KEY

Biology				
1. C	16. A	31. A	46. B	61. C
2. B	17. B	32. D	47. A	62. A
3. B	18. C	33. B	48. C	63. D
4. C	19. D	34. B	49. D	64. B
5. D	20. B	35. C	50. A	65. C
6. D	21. D	36. D	51. D	66. D
7. B	22. A	37. C	52. C	67. C
8. A	23. D	38. A	53. C	68. A
9. A	24. C	39. D	54. A	69. B
10. C	25. B	40. D	55. A	70. D
11. D	26. C	41. A	56. D	71. C
12. B	27. C	42. C	57. B	72. D
13. A	28. D	43. C	58. C	73. A
14. C	29. A	44. B	59. D	74. C
15. B	30. C	45. C	60. A	75. A

EXPLANATORY ANSWERS

1. **The correct answer is (C).**

   The cell is the smallest unit of life that can survive independently. The gene of a cell resides in the nucleus of the cell and can be considered an organelle, or part of the cellular machinery. An organ is composed of living cells.

2. **The correct answer is (B).**

   The mitochondria is the primary source of energy for the aerobic cell. The endoplasmic reticulum and Golgi apparatus use energy from the mitochondria to synthesize and store cellular products. The nucleus is primarily responsible for the storage of genetic information.

3. **The correct answer is (B).**

   By using a Punnett square, we see that two *Bb* individuals have a 1-in-4 (25%) chance of producing an offspring with blue (bb) eyes.

	B	*b*
B	*BB*	*Bb*
b	**Bb**	**bb**

4. **The correct answer is (C).**

   Hypertonic solutions have a greater salt, or electrolyte, concentration than do red blood cells. Therefore, water leaves blood cells and enters the hypertonic solution, causing the red blood cells to shrink. Both isotonic and iso-osmotic solutions will have no effect on the red blood cells. A hypotonic solution will cause water to enter the red blood cells because of their higher electrolyte concentration and cause the cells to swell.

5. **The correct answer is (D).**

   Copper is considered a trace element that is necessary for normal metabolism of the body. Sodium, potassium, and calcium are major elements vital to the healthy body.

6. **The correct answer is (D).**

	B	*B*
b	*Bb*	*Bb*
b	**Bb**	**Bb**

   A cross between a homozygous brown individual (*BB*) and a homozygous white individual (*bb*) will result in all offspring being brown heterozygous (*Bb*), as seen in the Punnett square.

7. **The correct answer is (B).**

   Vitamins A, D, E, and K are fat-soluble vitamins. All the B vitamins, as well as Vitamin C, are water-soluble vitamins.

8. **The correct answer is (A).**

Under basal conditions, the liver receives about 25 percent of the total cardiac output, whereas the brain and skeletal muscle receive about 15 percent. The bone is relatively nonvascularized and receives only 5 percent of the total blood flow.

9. **The correct answer is (A).**

Sodium is the most abundant electrolyte in extracellular fluid (~142 mEq/liter) with potassium the most abundant electrolyte (~141 mEq/liter) inside the cell (intracellular fluid). Both calcium (0–5 mEq/liter) and magnesium (3–58 mEq/liter) exist in relatively small amounts in the extracellular fluid.

10. **The correct answer is (C).**

The small intestine has the largest surface area and carries out most of the specialized transport mechanisms in the gastrointestinal tract. Very little absorption of nutrients occurs in the stomach or the large intestine, also referred to as the colon.

11. **The correct answer is (D).**

Long-chain (more than 10 carbons) fatty acids normally enter the circulatory system by way of the lymphatic system, packaged as chylomicrons. Short-chain fatty acids normally enter the circulatory system directly as free fatty acids.

12. **The correct answer is (B).**

See the explanation for Answer 9.

13. **The correct answer is (A).**

Scurvy is a disease resulting from a Vitamin C deficiency. Deficiencies in thiamine, niacin, and Vitamin D result in beriberi, pellagra, and rickets, respectively.

14. **The correct answer is (C).**

Squamous epithelium is normally associated with body surfaces, as a form of protection (i.e., skin). Epithelium associated with the kidney, lungs, and pancreas is more suited for secretory functions and is columnar or cuboidal in nature.

15. **The correct answer is (B).**

Chromatin is composed of DNA and protein and is found primarily in the nucleus.

16. **The correct answer is (A).**

Skeletal muscle fibers contract and relax in about 0.1 second. Cardiac muscle requires 1–5 seconds, whereas smooth muscle needs more than 3 seconds to contract and relax.

17. **The correct answer is (B).**

Saturated fats have all their carbon bonds saturated with hydrogens; thus, there are no double bonds. As the number of double bonds increases, the melting point of the fat decreases. Therefore, saturated fats are normally solids at room temperature, whereas unsaturated fats are liquids. Complete oxidation of 1 g. of fat yields about 9 calories, whereas 1 g. of carbohydrate yields about 4 calories.

18. The correct answer is (C).

Messenger RNA transfers genetic information from the nucleus by forming a complex with the ribosomes (composed largely of ribosomal RNA) of the endoplasmic reticulum in the cytoplasm. Transfer RNA carries amino acids to the messenger RNA-ribosome complex during protein synthesis.

19. The correct answer is (D).

Each mitotic division is a continuous process, with each stage merging imperceptibly into the next. For descriptive purposes, mitosis is divided into four successive stages: prophase, metaphase, anaphase, and telophase.

20. The correct answer is (B).

Since biological membranes are primarily a sandwich composed of a bimolecular layer of lipid with a layer of protein on both the inner and outer surfaces, lipid-soluble compounds diffuse through it faster than water-soluble compounds. For water-soluble compounds, the size of the molecule is the rate-limiting factor in diffusion.

21. The correct answer is (D).

Passive diffusion of a substance requires no energy (ATP) and will therefore not be affected by a metabolic inhibitor (cyanide). Passive diffusion also transfers uncharged (more lipid-soluble) molecules from a higher to a lower concentration.

22. The correct answer is (A).

A large sodium (Na^+) influx into the cell results in the resting potential (–50 mV) becoming more positive and thereby initiates the action potential. Potassium is already in very high concentration (~141 mEq/liter) intracellularly and will not enter the cell.

23. The correct answer is (D).

A large efflux of potassium (K^+) out of the cell results in a fall in electrical potential within the cell. Potassium, in high concentration intracellularly, easily leaves the cell, whereas sodium, in high concentration extracellularly, will not diffuse out of the cell rapidly.

24. The correct answer is (C).

The normal resting potential of –50 mV is established by the sodium-potassium pump of the cell, resulting in a high extracellular sodium concentration (~142 mEq/liter) and a high intracellular potassium concentration (A~141 mE~/liter). A negative resting potential is necessary to allow proper initiation of an action potential.

25. The correct answer is (B).

Insulin is a hormone that decreases blood glucose levels by increasing glucose uptake and storage by the cells. Pepsin, trypsin, and lactase are enzymes necessary for the proper digestion of nutrients.

26. The correct answer is (C).

The liver is the primary site of metabolism for the body and is responsible for detoxifying toxic agents in the blood. The lungs and kidneys both excrete these metabolized agents from the body. The pancreas does not directly metabolize toxic agents to any extent.

27. The correct answer is (C).

The kidneys remove waste products from the body.

28. The correct answer is (D).

All these processes are involved in the absorption of carbohydrates, amino acids, and fatty acids, as well as minerals and vitamins.

29. The correct answer is (A).

Bile salts are necessary for the proper digestion of fats in that they emulsify fat globules and render the end products of fat digestion soluble for more efficient absorption.

30. The correct answer is (C).

Glucose, fructose, and galactose are all simple sugars derived from hydrolytic cleavage of polysaccharides and double sugars. These simple sugars are then readily absorbed from the digestive tract. Glycogen is the storage form of glucose in the different cells of the body.

31. The correct answer is (A).

The brain does not store glucose as glycogen and must receive all its energy from glucose in the blood. Therefore, a rapid decrease in blood glucose immediately deprives the brain of the energy source it requires for normal function.

32. The correct answer is (D).

Vitamin A, or retinol, is converted in the retina to retinal, a light-sensitive pigment, necessary for night vision.

33. The correct answer is (B).

Both active transport and facilitated diffusion require carriers that combine with the transported substance. Passive diffusion involves the transfer of a substance from a region of higher concentration to one of lower concentration without a carrier.

34. The correct answer is (B).

Saturation of the carrier with the transferring substance in active transport and facilitated diffusion will lead to saturation kinetics. In addition, phagocytosis also has a maximum rate of transfer. Passive diffusion does not have any of these restrictions and normally proceeds at a rate proportional to the amount of substance present for transfer.

35. The correct answer is (C).

Mendel's first law, called the law of segregation, states that genes exist in individuals as pairs. The theory of recapitulation states that organisms tend to repeat, in the course of their evolutionary development, some of the corresponding stages of their evolutionary ancestors. Starling's law, also known as Starling's law of the heart, deals with regulation of the amount of blood pumped by the heart at a given time. The Watson-Crick model explains how the DNA molecule transfers information and undergoes replication.

36. The correct answer is (D).

About 56 percent of the adult human body is water (H_2O), with the rest of the body being primarily composed of organic molecules containing carbon. Therefore, of the four stated elements, calcium would be the least abundant in the human body.

37. The correct answer is (C).

Most species of animals and plants have chromosome numbers between 10–50. Humans have 46 chromosomes in each of their cells. Abnormalities in the chromosome number include Turner's syndrome (45 chromosomes) and Klinefelter's syndrome (47 chromosomes).

38. The correct answer is (A).

O-negative blood, by definition, contains no A, B, or Rh agglutinogens that would cause a transfusion reaction and possibly death for a blood recipient. Therefore, O-negative blood can be given to any individuals of the four major blood types.

39. The correct answer is (D).

Epinephrine is one of the neurotransmitters in the brain, especially in the thalamus and hypothalamus. Both norepinephrine and acetylcholine are transmitter substances known to be secreted by the autonomic nerves innervating smooth muscle. Cholecystokinin is a hormone secreted by the intestinal mucosa that causes specific contraction of the gallbladder.

40. The correct answer is (D).

Neutrophils, monocytes, eosinophils, and basophils are white blood cells produced by the bone marrow along with red blood cells. Lymphocytes are white blood cells that are produced by lymphoid tissue.

41. The correct answer is (A).

Actively acquired immunity depends upon the production of specific proteins, antibodies, that are released into the blood and tissue fluids in response to some foreign protein (an antigen) or vaccine. On the other hand, passively acquired immunity is a result of the injection of antibodies that have been produced in another individual or species. Natural immunity protects humans from infectious diseases associated with animals, such as canine distemper. Cellular immunity deals with the recognition and destruction of foreign, genetically different cells, and may be the cause of the rejection of transplanted organs.

42. The correct answer is (C).

Glomerular filtration is the process by which the kidney removes most of the waste products from the blood by pure filtration through the glomerular membrane. Hydrogen ions undergo tubular secretion into the glomerular filtrate, whereas substances such as glucose, amino acids, and potassium ions are actively reabsorbed by the tubular membrane. Sublimation is a physical change from the solid directly to the gaseous state, and does not apply to the kidney or any other organ.

43. The correct answer is (C).

Stimulation of the sympathetic nervous system increases the heart rate, sweating, and blood pressure and dilates the pupils of the eyes. Stimulation of the parasympathetic nervous system produces opposite effects, that is, decreases the heart rate, sweating and blood pressure, as well as constriction of the pupils.

44. The correct answer is (B).

During heavy exercise, glycogen in the muscle breaks down to lactic acid faster than lactic acid can be oxidized, resulting in lactic acid accumulation.

45. The correct answer is (C).

Meiosis occurs during the formation of eggs or sperm, where a pair of cell divisions result in gametes with only half the number of chromosomes (haploid) as the other cells of the body. When two gametes unite in fertilization, the fusion of their nuclei reconstitutes the diploid number of chromosomes.

46. The correct answer is (B).

The physical appearance of any individual with respect to a given inherited trait is known as his or her phenotype. In contrast, an individual's genetic constitution, usually expressed in symbols, is called his or her genotype. Both recessive and heterozygous traits are related more to genotype rather than phenotype.

47. The correct answer is (A).

Sickle-cell anemia is a condition where homozygous recessive genes are necessary for full development of the disease. If an individual has heterozygous recessive genes for the disease, that individual only shows sickle-cell trait, but not the fully developed disease. Both beriberi and pellagra are diseases associated with vitamin deficiencies. Hypertension is usually of unknown etiology.

48. The correct answer is (C).

Intense exercise and training of an athlete can result in a decreased respiratory rate and an increase in the size in muscle fibers. However, there will be no increase in the number of muscle fibers, since this does not change after birth.

49. The correct answer is (D).

Spermatogonia (diploid) grow into primary spermatocytes (diploid) and then secondary spermatocytes (diploid) after the first meiotic division. Secondary spermatocytes become spermatids (haploid) after the second meiotic division.

50. The correct answer is (A).

An individual with type A-negative blood can receive blood from A-negative or O-negative donors. Rh positive blood cannot be given, since a transfusion reaction would result. B- and AB-type bloods cannot be given for the same reason.

51. The correct answer is (D).

The appendix, wisdom teeth, and coccygeal vertebrae (tail bone) serve no useful purpose in humans; however, the pupils of the eyes are necessary for sight.

52. The correct answer is (C).

Graph C depicts a saturated reaction, as indicated by the initially straight lines for the product and substrate. The reaction proceeds to no substrate and all product, suggesting an irreversible reaction. Graph B indicates an unsaturated (curved lines) but irreversible (no substrate, all product after considerable time) reaction. Graph D represents an unsaturated reversible reaction, as shown by the initially curved line. This reaction also appears to be reversible, since the product and substrate appear to have reached an equilibrium. Thus, not all the substrate can be converted to product without some of the product reconverting to substrate.

53. **The correct answer is (C).**

The transport of oxygen and carbon dioxide in the blood depends largely on the amount of hemoglobin present in the red blood cell. Whole blood carries approximately 20 ml. of oxygen and 30–60 ml. of carbon dioxide per 100 ml. Plasma water carries only about 0.2–0.3 ml. of oxygen and carbon dioxide in each 100 ml. Plasma proteins carry essentially no oxygen.

54. **The correct answer is (A).**

Breeding between closely related individuals, commonly referred to as inbreeding, increases the proportion of homozygous individuals in a population, promoting the occurrence of double recessive traits of congenital anomalies. Some genetic disorders including muscular dystrophy and red-green color blindness are known to be sex-linked defective traits.

55. **The correct answer is (A).**

Beneficial associations or interactions between two species of animals include commensalism, protocooperation, and mutualism. Negative interactions between two species include amensalism, parasitism, and predation.

56. **The correct answer is (D).**

This question is similar to Question 52. Graph D shows unsaturated reaction characteristics (initially curved lines).

57. **The correct answer is (B).**

Albumin (~5 g./100 ml. of plasma) is the plasma protein most responsible for the osmotic pressure. Both fibrinogen and gammaglobulin are plasma proteins that contribute to the colloid osmotic pressure, but to a considerably lesser degree. Hemoglobin is a red pigment responsible for the transport of oxygen and carbon dioxide in the blood.

58. **The correct answer is (C).**

Only red blood cells carry hemoglobin, the substance responsible for oxygen and carbon dioxide transport.

59. **The correct answer is (D).**

Plasma cells, derived from lymphocytes, produce and secrete antibodies. Thrombocytes, important in initiating the clotting of blood, are formed by the fragmentation of giant cells, megakaryocytes, in the red bone marrow. Neutrophils are important in taking up bacteria and dead tissue cells by phagocytosis.

60. **The correct answer is (A).**

Cyanide is routinely employed as an inhibitor of enzymatic reactions. Therefore, treatment with cyanide will arrest the enzymatic reaction, and substrate will not be changed to product (Graph A).

61. The correct answer is (C).

The hemoglobin in the red blood cell has a high capacity for binding both oxygen and carbon dioxide. A lack of hemoglobin (anemia) results in a decreased capacity for oxygen and carbon dioxide transport.

62. The correct answer is (A).

Albumin (5 g./100 ml. of plasma) is approximately 2.5 times more abundant than globulin (2 g./100 ml. of plasma). Fibrinogen and immunoglobulins are present in small amounts compared to albumin.

63. The correct answer is (D).

Whereas decreased oxygen delivery to tissues (or a low blood oxygen concentration) will increase the number of red blood cells, increased carbon dioxide concentration will not. Changes in the number of red blood cells appear to be associated with changes in blood oxygen tension rather than in blood carbon dioxide tension.

64. The correct answer is (B).

Sweating, increased metabolism, and vasodilation of the blood vessels help transfer body heat to the surrounding environment. Increased muscle tone does not significantly increase heat loss.

65. The correct answer is (C).

Urea and creatinine normally pass through the kidney in the glomerular filtrate. Conversely, normally all the glucose in the glomerular filtrate is actively reabsorbed by the kidney in the normal individual. Glucose can be found in the urine when the blood glucose concentration is abnormally elevated (> 180 mg. percent), as in uncontrolled diabetes.

66. The correct answer is (D).

The reticular activating system is involved in the control of sleep, wakefulness, attentiveness, and behavior, but does not actively participate in regulating the volume of body fluids. The baroreceptors and vasomotor center of the brain work together to increase the flow of blood to the glomeruli of the kidneys, resulting in increased glomerular filtration and formation of urine. The osmoreceptors control the amount of water reabsorbed from the tubular filtrate of the kidneys by the secretion of antidiuretic hormone.

67. The correct answer is (C).

The axon and dendrites are components of the neuron. The dendrites constitute that part of the neuron specialized for receiving excitation, whereas the axon is the part specialized to distribute or conduct excitation away from the dendritic zone. Nerves are usually composed of collections of axons.

68. The correct answer is (A).

The rate of conduction increases as the diameter of the axon increases because there is less resistance to the action potential. Thus, larger nerve fibers have a faster rate of conduction than smaller ones. Myelin sheaths usually increase the rate of conduction by insulating the action potential on the axon from the external environment, again decreasing resistance.

69. The correct answer is (B).

The autonomic nervous system, composed of both sympathetic and parasympathetic nerves, is responsible for the involuntary activities of the body. Motor impulses reach the effector organ from the brain or spinal cord through a series of motor neurons comprising the corticospinal (pyramidal) and extracorticospinal (extrapyramidal).

70. The correct answer is (D).

Thyroxine is an iodinated derivative of the amino acid tyrosine. Other hormones derived from amino acids include melatonin and epinephrine. Prostaglandins are derivatives of 20-carbon unsaturated fatty acids, whereas estradiol and testosterone are derived from cholesterol.

71. The correct answer is (C).

A single muscle twitch is caused by an initiating action potential; however, there is a latent period after the generation of the action potential and initiation of the muscle twitch. After the latent period, the muscle contracts and then relaxes, followed by a refractory period in which the muscle will not respond to another action potential.

72. The correct answer is (D).

The nervous system provides instantaneous control of a body function, whereas hormones usually take a relatively long time (hours or days) to regulate a body function.

73. The correct answer is (A).

Progesterone is secreted by the corpus luteum and acts with estradiol to regulate the estrous and menstrual cycles. Vasopressin, secreted by the hypothalamus, stimulates the contraction of smooth muscles and has an antidiuretic action on kidney tubules. Aldosterone regulates metabolism of sodium and potassium and is secreted by the adrenal cortex.

74. The correct answer is (C).

The rods of the retina are responsible for peripheral, achromatic, and poor detail vision. Central, color, and detail vision is a function of the cones of the retina.

75. The correct answer is (A).

The rate of lymph flow is much slower (~100 ml./hr.) than blood flow (~5 liter/min.) in humans and most animal species.

Chapter 9: Chemistry

KEY POINTS TO REMEMBER
General Chemistry:

1) Basic concepts and tools

   a) Basic concepts:

      i) Physic property: can be measured/observed without changing the composition or identity of a substance

      ii) Chemical property: must carry out a chemical change in order to observe

      iii) Elements: cannot be separated into simpler substances by chemical means

      iv) Compounds: a substance composed of atoms of two or more elements chemically united in fixed proportions

      v) A substance can exist in the following three states: solid, liquid, and gas.

   b) Basic tools:

      i) SI units: K (temperature, absolute zero = –273.15°C), kg. (mass), m. (meter), s (time), J (energy) etc.

      ii) Significant figures:

         (1) Addition/subtraction: result must round off to the least precise measurement

         (2) Multiplication/division: result must round off to have the same significant numbers as the measurement having the least significant numbers

2) Atoms, molecules, and ions

   a) Atoms: usually made up of electrons, protons, and neutrons

   b) Molecules: an aggregate of at least two atoms held together by chemical forces

   c) Ions and ionic compounds

   d) Percent composition by mass: the percent by mass of each element in a compound

   e) Nomenclature of inorganic compounds: binary and ternary compounds; salts

3) Chemical equations: reactants → products

   a) Balanced chemical equations: obey the Law of Conservation of Mass; contain the same number of each kind of atom on each side of the equation

   b) Limiting reagent: the reactant used up first in a reaction

   c) Percent yield (% yield) $= \dfrac{\text{actual yield}}{\text{theoretical yield}} \times 100\%$

   d) Ionic equations: show dissolved ionic compounds in their free ions

     Spectator ions: ions not involved in the overall reaction

     Net ion equations: show only species that actually take part in the reaction

4) The periodic table

    a) Classification of elements: metals, nonmetals, and metalloids

    b) Atomic radius increases down a column and decreases across a row

    c) Metallic character of elements within a group increases down a column

5) Chemical bonds

    a) Valence electrons: electrons in the outermost shell

    b) Ionic bond: transfer of electrons from one atom to another

    c) Covalent bond: sharing electrons between two atoms

    d) Electronegativity: the ability of an atom to attract toward itself the electrons in a chemical bond. F is the most electronegative element.

    e) VSEPR models can predict the geometry of molecules based on repulsion of electron pairs; examples are, linear ($BeCl_2$), trigonal planar (BF_3), tetrahedral (CH_4), trigonal bipyramidal (PCl_5) and Octahedral (SF_6) structures

    f) Hybridization of atomic orbitals: the mixing of atomic orbitals in an atom to generate a set of new atomic orbitals

    g) Hydrogen bond: a special type of dipole-dipole interaction between the hydrogen atom in a polar bond, such as O–H and N–H. In general, only N, O, and F can form hydrogen bonding.

6) The gaseous state of matter

    a) Graham's law of gas diffusion or effusion: the diffusion or effusion rates of gases are inversely proportional to the square roots of their molar masses

    b) Boyle's law: $P_1V_1 = P_2V_2$ at constant n,T; n is the number of moles of gas present

    c) Charlie's law: $V \mu T$ at constant n, P

    d) Avogadro's law: $V \alpha n$ at constant P,T

    e) Ideal gas law: $PV = nRT$

    f) STP: the conditions of 0° C and 1 atm. One mole of gas occupies a volume of 22.4 liters at STP

    g) Dalton's law: the total pressure of a mixture of gases is the sum of the pressures that the each gas would exert if present alone

7) Solutions:

    a) Solute: the substance present in smaller amount. Solvent: the substance present in larger amount.

    b) In general: polar or ionic compounds dissolve in polar solvents; nonpolar compounds dissolve in nonpolar solvents (like dissolves like).

    c) Henry's law: the solubility of a gas in a liquid is proportional to the pressure of the gas over the solution.

    d) Molarity:

        M = (moles of solute)/(liter of solution)

        For dilution or mixing: $M_1V_1 + M_2V_2 + \ldots = M_{final}V_{final}$

e)   Mass percent concentration:

Mass percent = (g. solute) × 100/(total weight of solution);

ppm is part per million; ppb is part per billion.

f)   Normality:

N = (equivalents of solute)/(liter of solution)

For dilution or mixing: $N_1V_1 + N_2V_2 + \ldots = N_{final}V_{final}$

g)   Molality: m = (moles of solute)/(kg. solvent)

h)   Electrolyte: the water solution of this substance can conduct electricity.
Nonelectrolyte: the water solution of this substance cannot conduct electricity.

i)   Colligative properties of nonelectrolyte solutions: vapor pressure lowing, boiling pressure elevation, freezing pressure depression, and osmotic pressure

j)   Osmosis: diffusion of water into a higher concentrated solution through a semipermeable membrane. Osmosis pressure depends only on the molality of the solution.

8) Acids and bases

a)   Definitions

i)   Arrhenius acid: substances provide H^+ in aqueous solution; Arrhenius base: substances provide OH^- in aqueous solution

ii)   Brønsted-Lowry acid: a proton donor; Brønsted-Lowry base: a proton acceptor

iii)   Lewis acid: electron-pair acceptor; Lewis base: electron-pair donor

b) $K_w = [H^+][OH^-] = 1.0 \times 10^{-14}$ at 25°C

c)   pH = $-\log[H^+]$. Acidic solution: pH < 7; neutral solution: pH = 7;
Basic solution: pH > 7. pH + pOH = 14

d)   For a solution that contains a weak acid and its salt: pH = pK_a + log [base]/[acid]

e)   Acid-base reactions:

i)   strong acid + strong base → neutral solution

ii)   strong acid + weak base → acidic solution

iii)   weak acid + strong base → basic solution

iv)   weak acid + weak base → depends on relative values of K_a and K_b

f)   Buffer solutions: composed of a weak acid or base and its salt.

i)   Can resist small change in pH when small amount of acid or base is added

ii)   Selection of buffer solution: desired pH $\cong pK_a$ of the weak acid

iii)   Buffer range: pH range = $pK_a \pm 1$

9) Chemical equilibrium

    a) At equilibrium:

       Forward reaction rate = reverse reaction rate

    b) Equilibrium constant for a reaction:

       $aA + bB \longleftrightarrow cC + dD$

       Equilibrium constant: $K_{eq} = [C]^c[D]^d/[A]^a[B]^b$

    c) Le Chatelier's principle: if a stress is applied to a system in equilibrium, the system will respond in such a way as to relieve that stress and restore equilibrium under a new set of conditions

10) Oxidation-Reduction

    a) Oxidation number: electrons lost, gained, or unequally shared by an atom

    b) Oxidation: losing electrons → oxidation number increases → is a reducing agent

    c) Reduction: gaining electrons → oxidation number decreases → is an oxidizing agent

    d) Balancing oxidation-reduction equation: equalize loss and gain of electrons

11) Quantum chemistry

    a) Heisenberg Uncertainty Principle: it is not possible to know the position and the momentum of a particle simultaneously

    b) Quantum numbers:

      i) The principle quantum number n: the maximum number of electrons that n can hold is $2n^2$

      ii) The angular momentum quantum number l can have integer values from 0 to n–1; l = 0 → s orbital; l = 1 → p orbital

      iii) The magnetic quantum number (m_l) can have integer values from –1 to +1

      iv) The electron spin quantum number (m_s) can only have values of $-\dfrac{1}{2}$ and $+\dfrac{1}{2}$

    c) Pauli Exclusion Principle: no two electrons in an atom can have the same four quantum numbers

Organic Chemistry:

Basic organic compounds and functional groups:

1) Hydrocarbons: only contain carbon and hydrogen elements; can be divided into aliphatic hydrocarbons (no benzene group) and aromatic hydrocarbons (contain one or more benzene rings); aliphatic hydrocarbons can be further classified as alkanes, alkenes, and alkynes

    a) Alkanes: general formula C_nH_{2n+2}

    b) Alkenes: general formula C_nH_{2n}

    c) Alkynes: general formula of C_nH_{2n-2}

    d) Aromatic hydrocarbons

2) Alcohols: contain hydroxyl group, –OH; general formula: ROH.

    a) Classification: primary (1°), secondary (2°), or tertiary (3°) alcohols

    b) Oxidation: primary alcohols oxidize to aldehyde and further oxidize to carboxylic acid; secondary alcohols oxidize to ketones; tertiary alcohols normally cannot be oxidized.

    c) Carbon atoms exist in progressively higher stages of oxidation as follows: Alkanes → Alcohols → Aldehyde or Ketones → Carboxylic acids → Carbon dioxide. The carbon atoms in CH_4 and CO_2 represent the two extreme oxidation states of carbon, –4 and +4 respectively.

    d) Dehydration: forms alkenes or ethers

    e) Esterification: react with carboxylic acid to form esters. Alcohols lose –OH group and carboxylic acids lose –H group.

    f) Phenol: compounds having a hydroxyl group attached to an aromatic ring. The parent compound is phenol (C_6H_5OH). Phenol is a weak acid, more acidic than alcohols and water, but less acidic than acetic and carbonic acids.

3) Ethers: general formula of R–O–R'

4) Aldehydes and ketones: functional group is carbonyl group (–CO–). Aldehydes have the general formula of R–CHO. Ketones have the general formula of R–CO–R'.

    a) The carbon atom of the carbonyl group is sp^2 hybridized.

    b) Aldehydes can be oxidized to carboxylic acids, and give a positive Tollen's test (silver-mirror test), Fehling's test, and Benedict test. Normally, ketones cannot be oxidized and do not give positive tests.

    c) Aldehydes and ketones can be reduced to alcohols.

5) Carboxylic acids: functional group is the carboxyl group, –COOH; general formula is RCOOH

    a) Acid chlorides formation: carboxylic acids react with $SOCl_2$ or PCl_5

    b) Acetic acid can form Dimmer's to reduce its polarity.

    c) Ester formation: carboxylic acids react with alcohols

6) Esters: General formula for esters is RCOOR': R = H, alkyl, or aryl group; R' = alkyl or aryl group, but *not* a hydrogen; –COOR is the functional group.

    a) Hydrolysis: splitting of molecules through the addition of water

    b) Acid hydrolysis of esters: ester reacts with water to form an acid and an alcohol; catalyzed by strong acids or by certain enzymes

    c) Alkaline hydrolysis (Saponification): hydrolysis of ester by a strong base to form an alcohol and a salt

7) Amines: general formula is RNH_2 (primary amine), R_2NH (secondary amine), or R_3N (tertiary amine), where R = alkyl or aryl group; amines are organic bases.

8) Amides: general formula is $RCONH_2$, RCONHR, or $RCONR_2$; major reaction is hydrolysis.

Synthetic organic polymers and natural polymers in living systems:

1) Synthetic organic polymers: often called macromolecules; having high molar mass ranging into thousands and millions of grams

   a) Addition reactions and condensation reactions are two types of polymerization reactions

   b) Homopolymers: made from only one type of monomer

   c) Copolymerization: formation of polymer containing two or more different monomers

2) Carbohydrates: polyhydroxy ketones or substances that yield these compounds when hydrolyzed

   a) Classification: monosaccharides, disaccharides, and polysaccharides (or oligosaccharides)

   b) Monosaccharide: glucose is the most important. Glucose is a reducing sugar and gives a positive Tollen's test.

   c) Disaccharide: sucrose and lactose are two important disaccharides

   d) Polysaccharide: starch, cellulose, and glycogen are three important polysaccharides

3) Lipids: water insoluble, oily or greasy biochemical compounds that can be extracted from cells by nonpolar solvents

   a) Examples of lipids: fats, oils, steroids (cholesterol belongs to steroids)

4) Amino acids, polypeptides, and proteins

   a) Amino acids: general formula RNH_2COOH

      i) Classification: neutral (same number of amino and carboxyl groups), acidic (more carboxyl groups), and basic (more amino groups)

      ii) Glycine NH_2CH_2COOH is the simplest amino acid.

   b) Peptides: amino acid units joined through amide structures

   c) Proteins

      i) Primary structure: the number, kind, and sequence of amino acid units of the peptide chain or polypeptide chains

      ii) Secondary structure: regular, three-dimensional structure held together by hydrogen bonding between the oxygen of the carbonyl and –NH– group.

      α-helix and β-sheet are two examples.

      iii) Tertiary structure: refers to the distinctive and characteristic shape of a protein

5) Nucleic acids: DNA and RNA

   a) Chargaff's rule: the amount of A, G, C, T must satisfy A = T, C = G and A + G = C + T.

   b) Under normal conditions an A is paired with a T, and a G is paired with a C.

Answer Sheet

Chapter 9: Chemistry

1. Ⓐ Ⓑ Ⓒ Ⓓ   21. Ⓐ Ⓑ Ⓒ Ⓓ   41. Ⓐ Ⓑ Ⓒ Ⓓ   61. Ⓐ Ⓑ Ⓒ Ⓓ   81. Ⓐ Ⓑ Ⓒ Ⓓ

2. Ⓐ Ⓑ Ⓒ Ⓓ   22. Ⓐ Ⓑ Ⓒ Ⓓ   42. Ⓐ Ⓑ Ⓒ Ⓓ   62. Ⓐ Ⓑ Ⓒ Ⓓ   82. Ⓐ Ⓑ Ⓒ Ⓓ

3. Ⓐ Ⓑ Ⓒ Ⓓ   23. Ⓐ Ⓑ Ⓒ Ⓓ   43. Ⓐ Ⓑ Ⓒ Ⓓ   63. Ⓐ Ⓑ Ⓒ Ⓓ   83. Ⓐ Ⓑ Ⓒ Ⓓ

4. Ⓐ Ⓑ Ⓒ Ⓓ   24. Ⓐ Ⓑ Ⓒ Ⓓ   44. Ⓐ Ⓑ Ⓒ Ⓓ   64. Ⓐ Ⓑ Ⓒ Ⓓ   84. Ⓐ Ⓑ Ⓒ Ⓓ

5. Ⓐ Ⓑ Ⓒ Ⓓ   25. Ⓐ Ⓑ Ⓒ Ⓓ   45. Ⓐ Ⓑ Ⓒ Ⓓ   65. Ⓐ Ⓑ Ⓒ Ⓓ   85. Ⓐ Ⓑ Ⓒ Ⓓ

6. Ⓐ Ⓑ Ⓒ Ⓓ   26. Ⓐ Ⓑ Ⓒ Ⓓ   46. Ⓐ Ⓑ Ⓒ Ⓓ   66. Ⓐ Ⓑ Ⓒ Ⓓ   86. Ⓐ Ⓑ Ⓒ Ⓓ

7. Ⓐ Ⓑ Ⓒ Ⓓ   27. Ⓐ Ⓑ Ⓒ Ⓓ   47. Ⓐ Ⓑ Ⓒ Ⓓ   67. Ⓐ Ⓑ Ⓒ Ⓓ   87. Ⓐ Ⓑ Ⓒ Ⓓ

8. Ⓐ Ⓑ Ⓒ Ⓓ   28. Ⓐ Ⓑ Ⓒ Ⓓ   48. Ⓐ Ⓑ Ⓒ Ⓓ   68. Ⓐ Ⓑ Ⓒ Ⓓ   88. Ⓐ Ⓑ Ⓒ Ⓓ

9. Ⓐ Ⓑ Ⓒ Ⓓ   29. Ⓐ Ⓑ Ⓒ Ⓓ   49. Ⓐ Ⓑ Ⓒ Ⓓ   69. Ⓐ Ⓑ Ⓒ Ⓓ   89. Ⓐ Ⓑ Ⓒ Ⓓ

10. Ⓐ Ⓑ Ⓒ Ⓓ   30. Ⓐ Ⓑ Ⓒ Ⓓ   50. Ⓐ Ⓑ Ⓒ Ⓓ   70. Ⓐ Ⓑ Ⓒ Ⓓ   90. Ⓐ Ⓑ Ⓒ Ⓓ

11. Ⓐ Ⓑ Ⓒ Ⓓ   31. Ⓐ Ⓑ Ⓒ Ⓓ   51. Ⓐ Ⓑ Ⓒ Ⓓ   71. Ⓐ Ⓑ Ⓒ Ⓓ   91. Ⓐ Ⓑ Ⓒ Ⓓ

12. Ⓐ Ⓑ Ⓒ Ⓓ   32. Ⓐ Ⓑ Ⓒ Ⓓ   52. Ⓐ Ⓑ Ⓒ Ⓓ   72. Ⓐ Ⓑ Ⓒ Ⓓ   92. Ⓐ Ⓑ Ⓒ Ⓓ

13. Ⓐ Ⓑ Ⓒ Ⓓ   33. Ⓐ Ⓑ Ⓒ Ⓓ   53. Ⓐ Ⓑ Ⓒ Ⓓ   73. Ⓐ Ⓑ Ⓒ Ⓓ   93. Ⓐ Ⓑ Ⓒ Ⓓ

14. Ⓐ Ⓑ Ⓒ Ⓓ   34. Ⓐ Ⓑ Ⓒ Ⓓ   54. Ⓐ Ⓑ Ⓒ Ⓓ   74. Ⓐ Ⓑ Ⓒ Ⓓ   94. Ⓐ Ⓑ Ⓒ Ⓓ

15. Ⓐ Ⓑ Ⓒ Ⓓ   35. Ⓐ Ⓑ Ⓒ Ⓓ   55. Ⓐ Ⓑ Ⓒ Ⓓ   75. Ⓐ Ⓑ Ⓒ Ⓓ   95. Ⓐ Ⓑ Ⓒ Ⓓ

16. Ⓐ Ⓑ Ⓒ Ⓓ   36. Ⓐ Ⓑ Ⓒ Ⓓ   56. Ⓐ Ⓑ Ⓒ Ⓓ   76. Ⓐ Ⓑ Ⓒ Ⓓ   96. Ⓐ Ⓑ Ⓒ Ⓓ

17. Ⓐ Ⓑ Ⓒ Ⓓ   37. Ⓐ Ⓑ Ⓒ Ⓓ   57. Ⓐ Ⓑ Ⓒ Ⓓ   77. Ⓐ Ⓑ Ⓒ Ⓓ   97. Ⓐ Ⓑ Ⓒ Ⓓ

18. Ⓐ Ⓑ Ⓒ Ⓓ   38. Ⓐ Ⓑ Ⓒ Ⓓ   58. Ⓐ Ⓑ Ⓒ Ⓓ   78. Ⓐ Ⓑ Ⓒ Ⓓ   98. Ⓐ Ⓑ Ⓒ Ⓓ

19. Ⓐ Ⓑ Ⓒ Ⓓ   39. Ⓐ Ⓑ Ⓒ Ⓓ   59. Ⓐ Ⓑ Ⓒ Ⓓ   79. Ⓐ Ⓑ Ⓒ Ⓓ   99. Ⓐ Ⓑ Ⓒ Ⓓ

20. Ⓐ Ⓑ Ⓒ Ⓓ   40. Ⓐ Ⓑ Ⓒ Ⓓ   60. Ⓐ Ⓑ Ⓒ Ⓓ   80. Ⓐ Ⓑ Ⓒ Ⓓ   100. Ⓐ Ⓑ Ⓒ Ⓓ

Tear Here

Chemistry Practice Questions

100 QUESTIONS—50 MINUTES

Directions: Choose the best answer to each of the following questions.

1. Alkanes are NOT
   - (A) saturated compounds containing carbon and hydrogen.
   - (B) formed from sp^3 hybrid orbitals.
   - (C) arranged in a straight-chain sequence.
   - (D) of the general formula C_nH_{2n}.

2. Regarding phenol,
   - (A) a nitro substituent in the ortho position will lower the K_a.
   - (B) methyl substituent in the ortho position will lower the K_a.
   - (C) methyl substituent in the ortho position will increase the K_a.
   - (D) the OH substituent is a meta-directing group.

3. Which of the following is false?
   - (A) $pH = \dfrac{(\log 1)}{[H^+]}$
   - (B) $pH + pOH = 14$
   - (C) $(H^+)(OH^-) = 10^{-14}$
   - (D) $pH - pOH = 14$

4. Calculate the percentage of iron in hematite (Fe_2O_3), given the atomic weights of Fe = 56 and O = 16.
   - (A) 70%
   - (B) 2%
   - (C) 30%
   - (D) 49%

5. How many liters of hydrogen are required to produce 20 liters of ammonia, given the equation $3H_2 + N_2 \rightarrow 2NH_3$?
   - (A) 15 liters
   - (B) 30 liters
   - (C) $33\frac{1}{3}$ liters
   - (D) 40 liters

6. The volume occupied by the gram-molecular weight of a gas at 0°C and 760 mmHg is
   - (A) 1 liter.
   - (B) 22.4 liters.
   - (C) 32 liters.
   - (D) 100 liters.

7. Given the atomic weights of C = 12 and O = 16, what is the weight of 2 liters of carbon dioxide at standard temperature and pressure?
   - (A) 2 g.
   - (B) 4 g.
   - (C) 6 g.
   - (D) 8 g.

8. Which of the following hybrid orbitals would carbon form in acetylene?
   - (A) sp
   - (B) sp^2
   - (C) sp^3
   - (D) All of the above

9. Which of the following hybrid orbitals would methane and water both form?

    (A) sp

    (B) sp^2

    (C) sp^3

    (D) All of the above

10. The structural formula indicates all of the following EXCEPT the

    (A) number of atoms in a molecule.

    (B) gram-molecular volume.

    (C) types of atoms present.

    (D) arrangement of the atom.

11. Pick out the incorrect statement.

    (A) Organic compounds may exist as isomers.

    (B) Reactions involving organic compounds always proceed faster than those involving inorganic compounds.

    (C) Organic compounds are generally soluble in organic solvents.

    (D) Organic compounds decompose at relatively lower temperatures than inorganic compounds.

12. When the nucleus of an atom emits a beta particle, the atomic

    (A) weight decreases by 4.

    (B) weight increases by 1.

    (C) number increases by 1.

    (D) number stays the same.

13. The conversion of one element into another is termed

    (A) transformation.

    (B) disintegration.

    (C) transmutation.

    (D) emanation.

14. All the following are characteristics of gamma rays EXCEPT

    (A) high-energy X rays.

    (B) very short wavelength.

    (C) deflected by electric fields.

    (D) travel at the speed of light.

15. The energy released in nuclear reactions is due to

    (A) atomic fusion.

    (B) electron capture.

    (C) atomic fission.

    (D) both fusion and fission.

16. All of the following are alcohols EXCEPT

    (A) methanol.

    (B) ethanol.

    (C) glycerine.

    (D) sodium hydroxide.

17. Pick out the incorrect statement concerning hydrogen chloride gas.

    (A) It is lighter than air.

    (B) It has a pungent smell.

    (C) It is soluble in water.

    (D) It reacts with ammonia—forming ammonium chloride.

18. All of the following are halogens EXCEPT
    (A) bromine.
    (B) iodine.
    (C) chlorine.
    (D) turpentine.

19. The number of equivalents per mole for $HC_2H_3O_2$ is
    (A) 1
    (B) 2
    (C) 3
    (D) 4

20. Avogadro's law states that
    (A) under identical temperature and pressure, only certain gases contain the same number of molecules.
    (B) all gases contain different numbers of molecules, irrespective of pressure or temperature conditions.
    (C) only under equal volumes will all gases contain the same number of molecules.
    (D) under identical conditions of temperature and pressure, equal volumes of all gases contain the same number of molecules.

21. There are how many different configurations for 2-chlorobutane?
    (A) 8
    (B) 1
    (C) 2
    (D) 6

22. The absolute configuration of a chiral molecule may be assigned using the symbols
    (A) cis and trans.
    (B) R and S.
    (C) syn and anti.
    (D) alpha and beta.

23. Calculate the amount of sodium chloride crystals needed to supply 100 mg. of sodium ions (Na = 23, Cl = 35.5).
    (A) 180 mg.
    (B) 432 mg.
    (C) 355 mg.
    (D) 254 mg.

24. Calculate the concentration (in milligrams per milliliter) of a solution containing 2 mEq of sodium chloride per milliliter.
    (A) 585 mg./ml.
    (B) 355 mg./ml.
    (C) 230 mg./ml.
    (D) 117 mg./ml.

25. It has been ordered that Mr. Smith should receive 2 mEq of sodium chloride per kilogram of body weight. Since Mr. Smith weighs 60 kg., how much sodium chloride is needed?
    (A) 7 g.
    (B) 17 g.
    (C) 27 g.
    (D) 117 g.

26. Since the hospital stocks a 0.9% solution of sodium chloride, how much of this solution must be administered to Mr. Smith?

    (A) 777 ml.
    (B) 350 ml.
    (C) 3,500 ml.
    (D) 7,700 ml.

27. The pharmacy, however, could only supply a 0.45% solution of sodium chloride. How many liters of this solution must be given to Mr. Smith?

    (A) 1.5 liters
    (B) 3.0 liters
    (C) 4.5 liters
    (D) 6.0 liters

28. Electrolytes (e.g., sodium chloride) are important in establishing osmotic pressure; the unit used in measuring osmotic activity is the milliosmol. How many milliosmols of particles does 1 mole of sodium chloride present?

    (A) 1 mOsm
    (B) 2 mOsm
    (C) 3 mOsm
    (D) None of the above

29. Osmotic activity is a function of

    (A) electrolytes only.
    (B) nonelectrolytes only.
    (C) strong electrolytes only.
    (D) the total number of particles present in solution.

30. If one assumes complete dissociation, how many milliosmols of sodium chloride are in 100 ml. of a 0.9% solution?

    (A) 2 mOsm
    (B) 3 mOsm
    (C) 31 mOsm
    (D) 45 mOsm

31. Which of the following statements is false?

    (A) Hydrogen has one proton.
    (B) Hydrogen has one electron in the K shell.
    (C) Hydrogen has one neutron in its nucleus.
    (D) Hydrogen has an atomic number and an atomic weight of 1.

32. Beryllium has five neutrons and two electrons each in the K and L shell, respectively. Therefore, beryllium has an atomic weight of

    (A) 5 and an atomic number of 4.
    (B) 9 and an atomic number of 5.
    (C) 4 and an atomic number of 9.
    (D) 9 and an atomic number of 4.

33. The chemical symbol for mercury is Hg, whereas that for oxygen is O. If HgO is mercuric oxide, what is mercurous oxide?

    (A) HgO_2
    (B) Hg_2O
    (C) Hg_2O_3
    (D) Hg_3O_2

34. HNO_3 is the chemical formula for nitric acid; HNO_2 is the chemical formula for

(A) nitrous acid.

(B) nitronous acid.

(C) nitrate acid.

(D) nitrite acid.

35. The combination of an element A with an element B to form a new compound AB is called a synthetic reaction. The reverse of this reaction is called

(A) single replacement.

(B) synthesis.

(C) decomposition.

(D) double replacement.

36. Pick out the incorrect statement.

(A) Oxidation is associated with the loss of electrons.

(B) Oxidation-reduction reactions involve the loss and gain of electrons.

(C) The oxidized particle (atom) shows a decrease in valence number.

(D) Reduction involves the gain of electrons.

37. You are given the equation $ABC_3 \rightarrow AB + C_2$. The balanced equation is

(A) $2ABC_3 \rightarrow AB + 3C_2$

(B) $ABC_3 \rightarrow AB + C_2$

(C) $2ABC_3 \rightarrow 2AB + 3C_2$

(D) $3ABC_3 \rightarrow 3AB + 3C_2$

38. A molecule of oxygen contains two atoms of oxygen. How many atoms of oxygen does a molecule of ozone contain?

(A) Two

(B) Four

(C) One

(D) Three

39. Which statement is false?

(A) Oxygen burns by itself.

(B) Oxygen is an odorless and colorless gas.

(C) Oxygen supports combustion.

(D) Air contains about 20% oxygen.

40. Hydrogen peroxide decomposes to yield

(A) two molecules of water and two molecules of oxygen.

(B) one molecule of water and one molecule of oxygen.

(C) three molecules of water and two molecules of oxygen.

(D) two molecules of water and one molecule of oxygen.

41. A volumetric flask contains 5,000 ml. of water. What is the weight of this quantity of water?

(A) 50 g.

(B) 500 g.

(C) 5,000 g.

(D) 50,000 g.

42. Molarity (M) is best defined as moles of solute per

(A) kiloliter of solution.

(B) kilogram of solution.

(C) 100 ml. of solution.

(D) liter of solution.

43. A total of 40 g. of sodium hydroxide is dissolved in water to give a final volume of 400 ml. What is the molarity of this solution? (Na = 23, O = 16, H = 1)

(A) 0.25 *M*

(B) 2.5 *M*

(C) 25 *M*

(D) 0.1 *M*

44. How many moles of solute are there in 125 ml. of a 5 *M* solution of sodium hydroxide?

(A) 10.0 mol

(B) 3.40 mol

(C) 0.625 mol

(D) 6.25 mol

45. How much sodium hydroxide is there in 125 ml. of a 5 *M* solution of sodium hydroxide?

(A) 75.0 g.

(B) 62.5 g.

(C) 25.0 g.

(D) 80.5 g.

46. What is the molarity of 1 liter of pure water (H_2O) ?

(A) 55.5 *M*

(B) 18 *M*

(C) 19 *M*

(D) It cannot be determined.

47. All of the following are colligative properties of solutions EXCEPT the

(A) boiling point.

(B) vapor pressure.

(C) freezing point.

(D) specific gravity.

48. Given that the hydrogen ion concentration (moles per liter) of a solution is 1.0, what is its pH?

(A) 0

(B) 1

(C) 7

(D) 14

49. Given the same hydrogen ion concentration (in moles/liter) of 1.0, calculate the pH value of this solution.

(A) 0

(B) 1

(C) 7

(D) 14

50. The higher the pH of a solution, the

(A) lower the acidity.

(B) higher the hydrogen ion concentration.

(C) lower the basicity.

(D) stronger the acid.

51. Which of the following statements is false?

(A) Methane is important in addition reactions.

(B) Methane is explosive when combined with air.

(C) Methane is a major component of natural gas.

(D) Methane is commonly known as marsh gas.

52. All of the following are esters EXCEPT

(A) ethyl acetate.

(B) methyl salicylate.

(C) sodium formate.

(D) nitroglycerine.

53. Carbohydrates are compounds containing carbon, hydrogen, and oxygen. Which of the following is NOT a carbohydrate?

   (A) Glucose

   (B) Glyceryl stearate

   (C) Dextran

   (D) Cellulose

54. Pick out the nonsynthetic fiber.

   (A) Cellulose

   (B) Rayon

   (C) Orlon

   (D) Nylon

55. The uncertainty principle, which states that it is impossible to know with exactitude both the momentum and position of an electron simultaneously, is associated with

   (A) Heisenberg.

   (B) Planck.

   (C) de Broglie.

   (D) Bohr.

56. How many quantum numbers are necessary in order to define electronic wave functions?

   (A) 4

   (B) 3

   (C) 2

   (D) 1

57. Wolfgang Pauli's exclusion principle states that

   (A) no two electrons in an atom can have the same three quantum numbers.

   (B) no two electrons in an atom can have the same four quantum numbers.

   (C) no two electrons can have the same orbital.

   (D) any two electrons in an atom can have the same four quantum numbers.

58. The electronic distribution in the orbitals of an oxygen atom is

   (A) $1s^2 2s^4 2p^2$

   (B) $1s^2 2s^2 2p^4$

   (C) $1s^2 2s^2 2p^8$

   (D) $1s^2 2s^2 2p^6$

59. Carbon has 6 protons, and its atomic weight is 12. How many electrons and neutrons does it have?

   (A) 3 electrons, 9 neutrons

   (B) 6 electrons, 6 neutrons

   (C) 6 electrons, 12 neutrons

   (D) It cannot be determined.

60. Name the element with the electronic distribution $1s^2 2s^2 2p^2$.

   (A) Helium

   (B) Carbon

   (C) Beryllium

   (D) Oxygen

61. Isotopes are atoms of elements differing only in

   (A) valence.

   (B) the number of electrons.

   (C) chemical property.

   (D) mass.

62. Carbon-14 is a commonly used radioisotope in medical research. How many more neutrons does it have compared to natural carbon?

   (A) 2

   (B) 4

   (C) 6

   (D) 0

PART III: PCAT REVIEW AND PRACTICE QUESTIONS

63. Pick out the statement about gamma-ray decay that is false.

    (A) The number of protons does not change.

    (B) It results in a decrease of 4 units of atomic mass.

    (C) There is emission of photons.

    (D) The number of neutrons does not change.

64. Electromagnetic radiation has a wide spectrum of energies and wavelengths. The angstrom is widely used as a unit to measure wavelength. What does it equal in meters?

    (A) 1×10^{-15} m.

    (B) 1×10^{-9} m.

    (C) 1×10^{-10} m.

    (D) 1×10^{-11} m.

65. Pyrophosphoric acid is $H_4P_2O_7$. What does the prefix *pyro-* indicate?

    (A) Lowest oxidation state

    (B) Highest oxidation state

    (C) Highest hydrated form

    (D) Loss of water

66. Lead (Pb) has many industrial uses. Lead ion exists in two oxidation states, which are

    (A) divalent and tetravalent.

    (B) monovalent and trivalent.

    (C) divalent and pentavalent.

    (D) monovalent and divalent.

67. Plaster of paris is made by heating gypsum until it loses three fourths of its water of hydration. What alkaline-earth metal is found in gypsum and plaster of paris?

    (A) Phosphorus

    (B) Calcium

    (C) Magnesium

    (D) Barium

68. Hydrogen sulfide (H_2S) can be prepared by the action of an acid on any metallic sulfide. All of the following are characteristics of hydrogen sulfide EXCEPT

    (A) colorless gas.

    (B) denser than air.

    (C) nontoxic.

    (D) odor of rotten eggs.

69. What is the common name for the organic acid with the formula CH_3COOH?

    (A) Aqua fortis

    (B) Muriatic acid

    (C) Aqua regia

    (D) Vinegar

70. If table salt is sodium chloride, which of the following is the formula for baking soda?

    (A) $Na_2B_4O_7$

    (B) $MgSO_4$

    (C) Na_2CO_3

    (D) $NaHCO_3$

www.petersons.com   140   *Peterson's* ■ *PCAT Success*

71. HOCl is a more powerful oxidizing agent than chlorine. What is HOCl?

    (A) Tincture of iodine

    (B) Chloroform

    (C) Hypochlorous acid

    (D) Brine

72. Alkenes do NOT possess a(n)

    (A) pi bond.

    (B) alpha bond.

    (C) double bond.

    (D) sigma bond.

73. Amino acids are generally represented by the formula RNH_2COOH. What class of organic compounds is represented by $RCONH_2$?

    (A) Amides

    (B) Esters

    (C) Amines

    (D) Azides

74. In chemistry, the suffix -ase, as in lipase, denotes a(n)

    (A) carboxyl group.

    (B) base.

    (C) enzyme.

    (D) sugar.

75. A primary alcohol has at least two hydrogens attached to the alcohol carbon. A tertiary alcohol has

    (A) no hydrogens attached to the alcohol carbon.

    (B) only hydrogen attached to the alcohol carbon.

    (C) three hydrogens attached to the alcohol carbon.

    (D) only one hydrogen attached to the alcohol carbon.

76. Which of the formulas below is methyl vinyl ketone?

    (A) $CH_3OCH_2CH = CH_2$

    (B) $CH_3COCH = CH_2$

    (C) $CH_3CH_2CH_2 = COOH$

    (D) $CH_3CH_2COCH = CH_2$

77. The incorrect way of naming an organic acid is by

    (A) using the hydrocarbon name of the longest chain.

    (B) designating the carboxyl carbon as carbon number 1.

    (C) changing the suffix from -ane to -anoic.

    (D) changing the suffix from -ane to -ol.

78. Name the hydrocarbon, $CH_3(CH_2)_8CH_3$.

    (A) Nonane

    (B) Octane

    (C) Undecane

    (D) Decane

79. Pick out the incorrect statement.

    (A) Atoms connected by single bonds rotate around the bond.

    (B) Atoms in double bonds are not free to rotate.

    (C) Atoms in a ring are free to rotate around their bonds.

    (D) Atoms in triple bonds are not free to rotate.

80. Pick out the incorrect statement.

    (A) The stability of a carbonium ion is increased by charge dispersal.

    (B) A primary carbonium ion forms more easily than a tertiary carbonium ion.

    (C) The carbon atom in a carbonium ion has only 6 electrons.

    (D) Carbonium ions can be classified as primary, secondary, or tertiary.

81. With regard to benzene, which one of the following statements is incorrect?

    (A) It is a flat (planar) molecule.

    (B) It has the formula C_6H_6.

    (C) It is a symmetrical molecule.

    (D) It has a bond angle of 150°.

82. With regard to the carbonyl carbons of aldehydes and ketones, which one of the following statements is false?

    (A) They usually have a bond angle of 120°.

    (B) They are oriented such that carbon and oxygen are joined by a double bond.

    (C) They are sp^2 hybridized and not planar.

    (D) They are connected to three other atoms by sigma bonds.

83. Nucleophilic substitution is commonly encountered in organic chemistry. Select the one statement below that is correct, concerning nucleophilic displacement.

    (A) Amines are more reactive than amides.

    (B) Acid chlorides are more reactive than alkyl chloride.

    (C) Ethers are more reactive than esters.

    (D) Saturated carbons are more reactive than acyl carbon.

84. Glycols are

    (A) alcohols containing two hydroxyl groups.

    (B) alcohols without any hydroxyl group.

    (C) aldehydes containing two hydroxyl groups.

    (D) ketones containing two hydroxyl groups.

85. The Grignard reagent is very useful in organic chemistry. Pick out the one incorrect statement about it.

    (A) Its general name is alkylmagnesium halide.

    (B) The magnesium-halogen bond is covalent.

    (C) The carbon-magnesium bond is considered covalent.

    (D) Its general formula is RMgX.

86. Which is the correct statement?

    (A) Optically inactive reactants yield optically active products.

    (B) Optically active products are the result of optically inactive reactants.

    (C) Optically inactive reactants yield optically inactive products.

    (D) The preparation of dissymmetric compounds from symmetric reactants yields no racemic modification.

87. If CH_4 is methane, what is CH_2?

    (A) Methanol

    (B) Mesyl

    (C) Methyl

    (D) Methylene

88. The Diels-Alder reaction does NOT involve
    (A) a diene and a dienophile.
    (B) a product that is six-membered.
    (C) $\alpha\beta$-unsaturated carbonyl compounds.
    (D) electron-releasing groups in the dienophile.

89. Disaccharides are composed of two monosaccharide units. Which of the following is NOT a disaccharide?
    (A) Amylose
    (B) Lactose
    (C) Maltose
    (D) Sucrose

90. Which of the following amino acids is simplest in structure?
    (A) Arginine
    (B) Tyrosine
    (C) Glycine
    (D) Methionine

91. Aryl halides are compounds containing halogen attached
    (A) to a side chain of an aromatic ring.
    (B) directly to an aromatic ring.
    (C) directly to a cyclic alkane.
    (D) to an alkene.

92. Ethylene oxide is best described as an
    (A) alkane.
    (B) alkene.
    (C) aldehyde.
    (D) epoxide.

93. Amines may have all of the following formulas EXCEPT
    (A) RNH_2
    (B) R_3N
    (C) RNH
    (D) R_2NH

94. Absolute alcohol is
    (A) a mixture of fifty parts of alcohol to water.
    (B) 80% alcohol.
    (C) water-free alcohol.
    (D) wood alcohol.

95. Two aromatic rings sharing a pair of carbon atoms are called fused-ring hydrocarbons. The simplest member of this family of compounds is
    (A) naphthalene.
    (B) phenanthrene.
    (C) benzene.
    (D) anthracene.

96. CH_3OH is usually known as
    (A) menthone.
    (B) methanol.
    (C) menthol.
    (D) mesitol.

97. All the following describes Tollen's reagent EXCEPT
    (A) reduction of silver ion to free silver.
    (B) oxidation of an aldehyde.
    (C) reduction of an acid to aldehyde.
    (D) silver ammonia ion.

98. In forming ammonia, nitrogen uses

(A) sp orbitals.

(B) sp^1 orbitals.

(C) sp^2 orbitals.

(D) sp^3 orbitals.

---

99. An acid chloride can be prepared by substitution of the hydroxyl group of a carboxylic acid. The following reagents are commonly used to prepare acid chlorides EXCEPT

(A) thionyl chloride.

(B) ethyl chloride.

(C) phosphorus trichloride.

(D) phosphorus pentachloride.

100. Which is the incorrect statement?

(A) Sucrose is a reducing sugar.

(B) All monosaccharides are reducing sugars.

(C) Glucose is a monosaccharide.

(D) Glucose is a reducing sugar.

ANSWER KEY

Chemistry				
1. D	21. C	41. C	61. D	81. D
2. B	22. B	42. D	62. A	82. C
3. B	23. D	43. B	63. B	83. B
4. A	24. D	44. C	64. C	84. A
5. B	25. A	45. C	65. D	85. B
6. B	26. A	46. A	66. A	86. C
7. B	27. A	47. D	67. B	87. D
8. A	28. B	48. A	68. C	88. D
9. C	29. D	49. D	69. D	89. A
10. B	30. C	50. A	70. D	90. C
11. B	31. C	51. A	71. C	91. B
12. C	32. D	52. C	72. B	92. D
13. C	33. B	53. B	73. A	93. C
14. C	34. A	54. A	74. C	94. C
15. D	35. C	55. A	75. A	95. A
16. D	36. C	56. A	76. B	96. B
17. A	37. C	57. B	77. D	97. C
18. D	38. D	58. B	78. D	98. D
19. A	39. A	59. B	79. C	99. B
20. D	40. D	60. B	80. B	100. A

EXPLANATORY ANSWERS

1. **The correct answer is (D).**

    Alkanes are saturated hydrocarbons containing only carbon and hydrogen. They are usually straight-chained compounds and the carbon atom utilizes four sp^3 hybrid orbitals, forming a tetrahedral arrangement. Each bond angle is 109.5°, and the general formula is C_nH_{2n+2}; for example, when there is one C atom, then there are four H atoms, as in methane. Alkenes have the general formula C_nH_{2n}.

2. **The correct answer is (B).**

    With regard to phenol, electron-releasing substituents (e.g., $-CH_3$) will decrease its acidity and lower the K_a. An electron-attracting substituent (e.g., $-NO_2$) will withdraw the ring electrons, relatively, and increase the acidity of phenol, resulting in a higher K_a. Thus, a nitro substituent in the ortho position will increase the K_a, whereas a methyl substituent in the same position would lower the K_a. Furthermore, the $-OH$ substituent is strongly ortho and para directing.

3. **The correct answer is (B).**

    Using the pH concept, we have $pH = -\log[H^+] = \log\left[\dfrac{1}{[H^+]}\right]$.

    Furthermore, $pOH = \log\left[\dfrac{1}{[OH^-]}\right]$, and $[H^+][OH^-]$ equals 10^{-14}.

    From these relations, $pH + pOH = 14$.

4. **The correct answer is (A).**

    Hematite (Fe_2O_3) has a molecular weight of 160. The percentage of elemental iron in hematite is given as follows:

    $$\frac{2Fe}{Fe_2O_3} = \frac{2(56)}{160} \times 100\%$$
    $$= 70\%$$

    Note that there are two atoms of iron in Fe_2O_3.

5. **The correct answer is (B).**

    $$3H_2 \quad + \quad N_2 \quad \rightarrow \quad 2NH_3$$
    (3 liters)   (1 liter)   (2 liters)

    Setting up a direct proportion, that is,

    $$\frac{2 \text{ liters of } NH_3}{2 \text{ liters of } H_2} = \frac{20 \text{ liters of } NH_3}{x \text{ liters of } H_2}$$

    and solving for x will give an answer of 30 liters.

6. **The correct answer is (B).**

The volume occupied by the gram-molecular weight of a gas under standard temperature and pressure conditions (i.e., 0°C and 760 mmHg) is called the gram-molecular volume. Hence, 1 mole of any gas under these conditions will occupy a volume of 22.4 liters. Be aware that 1 mole of the same gas may occupy a different volume at some other combination of temperature and pressure.

7. **The correct answer is (B).**

The molecular weight of CO_2 is 44 g. (i.e., 12 + 32). Thus, the gram-molecular weight of CO_2 is 44 g., which occupies 22.4 liters at standard temperature and pressure. Therefore, the weight of 1 liter of

CO_2 equals $\dfrac{(44\ g)}{(22.4\ liters)}$ = 1.9 g. Since there are 2 liters of CO_2, the weight is 4 g.

8. **The correct answer is (A).**

In acetylene, carbon forms two *sp* hybrid orbitals and thus enables itself to bind to two hydrogen atoms in a sigma bond. The carbon-carbon triple bond, however, is made up of one sigma bond and two pi bonds.

9. **The correct answer is (C).**

The carbon in methane (CH_4) and the oxygen in water (H_2O) both form sp^3 hybrid orbitals. For carbon, the sp^3 hybridization results in four hybrid orbitals in which the axes are directed toward the corners of a tetrahedron. In the formation of water, oxygen bonds with two hydrogen atoms via its two unpaired electrons. The water molecule still has a tetrahedral shape; two corners are occupied by hydrogen atoms and the rest is occupied by the unshared pairs of electrons.

10. **The correct answer is (B).**

In chemistry, the structural formula (e.g., $C_6H_{12}O_6$) reveals the numbers and types of atoms present in a molecule. In general, if not always, the arrangement of the different atoms can also be deduced from an examination of the structural formula. However, the structural formula of a molecule bears no relationship to the gram-molecular volume occupied by the gram-molecular weight of a gas under standard conditions.

11. **The correct answer is (B).**

A knowledge of the chemical and physical properties of organic and inorganic compounds is important in understanding their chemical behavior. Organic compounds do exist as isomers and decompose upon heating at lower temperatures. They are also soluble in other organic solvents; that is, like dissolves like. However, organic compounds do not react with each other faster than inorganic compounds would.

12. **The correct answer is (C).**

In radioactive disintegration, the emission of a beta particle does not change the atomic weight of the nucleus emitting the beta particle. This is due to the fact that the weight of a beta particle is extremely small. However, the atomic number increases by 1 and is thought to be the result of the breakdown of a neutron to a proton and an electron (beta particle). An alpha particle is a helium nucleus, and its emission, in contrast to that of a beta particle, results in a decrease of 4 units of atomic weight and 2 units of atomic number.

13. The correct answer is (C).

The artificial conversion of one element into another (e.g., nitrogen into oxygen) is termed transmutation. Radioactive decay can occur spontaneously, resulting in the disintegration of the parent nucleus, with the consequent production of one or more daughter nuclei. This process is usually accompanied by the emanation (i.e., emission) of gamma rays. *Transformation* is a nonspecific term for changes in physical form.

14. The correct answer is (C).

Gamma rays are high-energy X rays of very short wavelength that travel with the speed of light. Compared to alpha and beta rays, gamma rays are the most penetrating of the radiations emitted by radioactive compounds. Since they have no electrical charge, magnetic or electrical fields do not affect their path.

15. The correct answer is (D).

Atomic fusion is the process of combining atoms to form elements of higher atomic weight. Frequently, tremendous energy is released during this process. Atomic fission is the process of splitting an atomic nucleus, which also results in the release of large amounts of energy. The process of electron capture results from the conversion of an orbital electron to a neutron, and the energy therein is negligible compared to that of atomic fusion and fission.

16. The correct answer is (D).

Alcohols have the general formula ROH. While methanol and ethanol are the simplest and most easily recognized alcohols, glycerine is also an alcohol, even though it has three hydroxyl groups. Glycerine (or glycerol) is thus a polyalcohol and is widely used in pharmaceutical manufacturing. Sodium hydroxide (NaOH) is a base and not an alcohol. Remember that alcohols are organic compounds in which the hydroxyl group has been substituted for one or more hydrogen atoms in a hydrocarbon.

17. The correct answer is (A).

Hydrogen chloride gas has a pungent smell, is extremely soluble in water, and reacts with ammonia to form white fumes of ammonium chloride. It is a colorless gas, but is not lighter than air. The density of the gas is greater than 1 g./cm.^{3} and is about 25% heavier than air.

18. The correct answer is (D).

The halogen elements are fluorine, chlorine, bromine, iodine, and astatine. They comprise group VIIA of the periodic table. Note that these elements end in the suffix *-ine*; however, this does not mean that turpentine or nicotine belong to the halogen family.

19. The correct answer is (A).

It can be stated that 1 Eq of any chemical is that quantity that is equivalent to 1 mole of replaceable hydrogen ions in an acid-base reaction. Thus, 1 mole of HCl contains 1 mole of replaceable hydrogen, and thus HCl has 1 Eq/mole. $HC_2H_3O_2$ is the formula for acetic acid, CH_3COOH. Clearly, only one hydrogen ionizes, and therefore acetic acid has 1 Eq/mole.

20. The correct answer is (D).

Avogadro's law determines the relation between the properties of gases. In essence, it states that equal volumes of different gases at the same temperature and pressure contain the same number of molecules. Hence, if one keeps the temperature and pressure constant, the volume of any gas is proportional to its mass, and therefore to the number of gas molecules. Note that Charles' law states that the volume of a gas is directly proportional to the absolute temperature, provided that pressure remains constant. Boyle's law relates the pressure and volume of a gas at constant temperature.

21. The correct answer is (C).

There is one chiral center, and thus 2 possible isomers or 2 configurations.

22. The correct answer is (B).

R from the Latin *rectus*, meaning right and S from the Latin *sinister*, meaning left.

23. The correct answer is (D).

If one assumes complete ionization, 58.5 mg. of sodium chloride will supply 23 mg. of sodium ions. Similarly, to give 100 mg. of sodium ions, it is required to supply $\frac{(100 \times 58.5)}{23} = 254$ mg. of sodium chloride crystals.

24. The correct answer is (D).

One mEq of sodium chloride is equal to its gram-equivalent weight divided by 1000. Hence, 1 mEq of sodium chloride equals 58.5 mg of sodium chloride and 2 mEq equals 117 mg. The concentration of this solution is 117 mg/ml.

25. The correct answer is (A).

The milliequivalent is used primarily by the health profession to express the concentration of electrolytes in solution. Since Mr. Smith weighs 60 kg., he should receive 2 × 60 mEq of sodium chloride. One mEq of sodium chloride equals 58.5 mg of salt. Therefore, Mr. Smith requires 2 × 60 × 58.5 mg. of sodium chloride. The answer is 7,020 mg., or 7 g.

26. The correct answer is (A).

Percent (%) means parts per hundred on a weight basis. Hence, a 0.9% solution translates to 0.9 g. of sodium chloride per 100 ml. of solution. Mr. Smith requires 7 g., which is $\frac{(7 \times 100 \text{ ml.})}{0.9}$ of solution. This comes out to 777 ml. of a 0.9% solution of sodium chloride.

27. The correct answer is (A).

The pharmacist must be well versed with the different units used to express the strength or concentration of a particular drug in solution. This problem relates to a solution of sodium chloride that is half the strength ordered. Hence, twice the volume must be supplied to give the same amount of sodium chloride ordered, that is, 777 ml × . 2 = 1.5 liters.

28. The correct answer is (B).

Osmotic pressure is directly affected by the total number of particles in solution. If one assumes complete dissociation, 1 mole of sodium chloride is composed of 2 mOsm of total particles (i.e., Na^+ and Cl^-).

29. The correct answer is (D).

Osmotic activity is a function of the total number of particles present in a given solution, be they electrolytes or nonelectrolytes. Electrolytes, in general, will dissociate into their component ions, and hence the number of particles in solution will increase.

30. The correct answer is (C).

This question illustrates the need to convert different units to arrive at the answer. One millimole of sodium chloride is equal to 2 mOsm of the salt. One millimole of sodium chloride is 58.5 mg. Since a 0.9% solution has 0.9 g. (or 900 mg.) of sodium chloride per 100 ml. of solution, 900 mg. of this sodium chloride is equal to $\frac{900}{58.5}$ or 15.4 mmole of sodium chloride. Now, since 1 mmole of sodium chloride is equal to 2 mOsm, 15.4 mmole equals 15.4×2 mOsm of sodium chloride. The answer is 31 mOsm.

31. The correct answer is (C).

Hydrogen has an atomic number and an atomic weight of 1. Hence, it has one proton and one electron, which reside in the nucleus and *K* shell, respectively. Hydrogen does not have a neutron. The hydrogen isotopes deuterium and tritium have one and two neutrons in the nucleus, respectively.

32. The correct answer is (D).

This problem relates to the concept of atomic weight and atomic number. The total number of protons equals the number of electrons in the shells. Beryllium has four electrons, and therefore four protons. The total number of protons equals the atomic number, and therefore beryllium has an atomic number of 4. The total number of protons and neutrons comprises the atomic weight of the element. Beryllium has an atomic weight of 9, since it has five neutrons and four protons.

33. The correct answer is (B).

Mercury forms bivalent mercuric (Hg^{2+}) and bivalent mercurous (Hg_2^{2+}) compounds, even though mercury has a valence of 2 and 1, respectively. Mercurous oxide is Hg_2O. Hg_2O_3, Hg_3O_2, and HgO_2 compounds are unknown.

34. The correct answer is (A).

HNO_2 is nitrous acid. Nitronous acid, nitrate acid, and nitrite acid do not exist.

35. The correct answer is (C).

The reverse of synthesis is decomposition, that is, the breakdown of a compound AB to yield an element A and an element B.

36. The correct answer is (C).

When a particle is oxidized, it loses electrons. Therefore, oxidation is associated with electron loss. Conversely, reduction is associated with electron gain. Since oxidation and reduction processes occur simultaneously, loss and/or gain of electrons is to be expected. An oxidized particle therefore loses its (valence) electrons, which results in an increase in valence number.

37. The correct answer is (C).

This is an exercise in the law of conservation of matter. Examination of the equation will show that the number of molecules of the reactants must equal the number of molecules of the products, that is,

$$2ABC_3 \quad \rightarrow \quad 2AB + 3C_2$$

Reactant	=	Product
2A		2A
2B		2B
6C		6C

38. The correct answer is (D).

The oxygen molecule is diatomic (O_2). Ozone is a triatomic molecule (O_3) of oxygen; its properties are different from those of oxygen.

39. The correct answer is (A).

It is common knowledge that oxygen gas is combustible; however, it cannot be overemphasized that oxygen *supports* combustion and does not burn by itself. Its lack of odor and color does not help in its quick identification.

40. The correct answer is (D).

Hydrogen peroxide is H_2O_2. The word *peroxide* means that it contains one more oxygen atom than would normally be expected. Water (H_2O) is the simplest molecule formed between the atoms of oxygen and hydrogen. Two molecules of hydrogen peroxide decompose via the following reaction, yielding two molecules of water and one molecule of oxygen: $2H_2O_2 \rightarrow 2H_2O + O_2$

41. The correct answer is (C).

This problem deals with the concept of density. Since the gram is defined as the mass of 1 cm³ (approximately 1 ml.) of water at 4°C, water has a density of 1 g./ml.; 5,000 ml. of water weigh 5,000 g.

42. The correct answer is (D).

The student is expected to be familiar with the different units used in expressing the quantity of a given solute in a quantity of solvent or total solution. Molarity (*M*) is defined as the number of moles of solute per liter of solution. In contrast, molality is the number of moles of solute in 1 kg of solvent. You should also be aware that normality (*N*) is defined as the number of equivalents of solute per liter of solution.

43. The correct answer is (B).

The molecular weight of NaOH is 40. Hence, 40 g. of NaOH are equivalent to 1 mole of NaOH. Molarity is defined as the number of moles of solute per liter of solution. Therefore, 1 mole of NaOH dissolved in 1 liter of solution is a 1 M solution. Dissolving 1 mole in 400 ml. would give a higher molarity, that is, an increase by a factor of 2.5.

44. The correct answer is (C).

If you are still unclear about moles and molarity by the time you get to this question, a review is required. One mole of sodium hydroxide equals 40 g. dissolved in 1 liter of solution. A 5 M (molar) solution would mean 5 × 40 g. of sodium hydroxide dissolved in 1 liter of solution. Hence, 125 ml. of this solution would contain (125 × 5 × 40)/1,000 of sodium hydroxide. The number of moles would now be easy to calculate: Just divide (125 × 5 × 40) g. /1,000 by 40 g./mole. The answer is 0.625 mole.

45. The correct answer is (C).

Since 125 ml of a 5 M solution contains 0.625 mole of sodium hydroxide, then 0.625 mole × 40 g./mole of sodium hydroxide yields 25 g. of this base.

46. The correct answer is (A).

A liter of pure water weighs 1 kg., if one assumes that water has a density of 1 g./ml. The molecular weight of water is 18 g./mole. One liter of pure water, therefore, contains $\dfrac{1,000 \text{ g.}}{18 \text{ g. / mole}}$ or 55.5 moles; 55.5 moles of water in a solution represents a molarity of 55.5.

47. The correct answer is (D).

Colligative properties of solutions depend on the amount and concentration of the solute(s) in the solution. Hence boiling point, vapor pressure, and freezing point are all colligative properties. Specific gravity, which compares the weights of substances to that of water, is not a colligative property.

48. The correct answer is (A).

Acid and base strengths are frequently expressed by pH values. The pH value of any number is defined as the negative logarithm (base 10) of that number; that is, if $x = 10^n$, then $\log x = n$ and the pH of x is $-n$. Since pH = $-\log[H^+]$ = $-\log[1]$, pH = 0. Note that a pH of 0 is not neutral. A pH of 7 represents neutrality.

49. The correct answer is (D).

Since pOH + pH = 14 and pH = 0, pOH equals 14. This would represent a very basic (strongly alkaline) solution.

50. The correct answer is (A).

As indicated before, the pH value gives some idea of the strength of an acid or base. The higher the pH value, the lower the hydrogen ion concentration. A higher pH means that the substance is less acidic and more basic.

51. The correct answer is (A).

Methane (CH_4) is the simplest saturated hydrocarbon of the alkane series. It is explosive when mixed with air, is the active component of natural gas, and is otherwise called marsh gas. Owing to its saturated character, methane is not important in addition reactions, but it will undergo substitution reactions.

52. The correct answer is (C).

Esters have the general formula RCOOR. Ethyl acetate is $C_2H_5COOCH_3$. Nitroglycerine and methyl salicylate are both esters. Sodium formate (NaCOOH) is the salt of an organic acid and is therefore not an ester.

53. The correct answer is (B).

Glucose is a monosaccharide. Dextran and cellulose are polysaccharides. Glyceryl stearate is a fatty acid and is widely employed in making soaps, for example, sodium stearate.

54. The correct answer is (A).

Rayon, nylon, and Orlon are all synthetic fibers. Nylon is a synthetic protein, Orlon is a polyester fiber, and rayon is regenerated cellulose; however, cellulose is a nonsynthetic fiber.

55. The correct answer is (A).

Werner Heisenberg showed that when one attempts to simultaneously determine the position and momentum of an electron, an unavoidable uncertainty in both these parameters is created that cannot be resolved. Louis de Broglie advanced the hypothesis that electrons have wavelike characteristics, Planck is responsible for the foundations of quantum theory, and Bohr is known for his electronic theory of the atom.

56. The correct answer is (A).

Four quantum numbers are necessary in order to fully characterize the electronic wave functions; these are n (the principle quantum number), 1 (the azimuthal quantum number), m (the magnetic quantum number), and s (the spin quantum number).

57. The correct answer is (B).

Pauli's exclusion principle clearly demonstrates that an atom cannot exist in a state where two electrons in the same orbital have the same four quantum numbers. This principle is important when more and more electrons are added to the orbitals of the atoms in the periodic table.

58. The correct answer is (B).

The student is expected to remember the atomic numbers of the first ten elements in the periodic table. Oxygen has eight electrons and its orbitals are filled according to a $1s^2 2s^2 2p^4$ electronic configuration. You should remember the minimum (or maximum) number of electrons that can occupy any orbital. These $s, p, d,$ and f orbitals can be completely filled by 2, 6, 10, and 14 electrons, respectively.

59. The correct answer is (B).

Carbon has 6 protons and, therefore, 6 electrons; however, its atomic weight is 12; that is, it has 6 protons and 6 neutrons. Hence, carbon has 6 protons, 6 electrons, and 6 neutrons. Remember that the atomic number is equal to the number of protons (or electrons) and that the atomic weight is the number of protons *and* neutrons in the nucleus.

60.   The correct answer is (B).

The $1s^2 2s^2 2p^2$ electronic distribution translates to 6 orbital electrons. Hence, this element has 6 electrons and therefore 6 protons. Carbon has 6 protons and 6 electrons. Beryllium has 4 electrons, helium has 2, and oxygen has 8. The element in question is carbon.

61.   The correct answer is (D).

Isotopes are atoms of elements having the same number of electrons, the same chemical characteristics, and the same valence. However, isotopes differ in their mass, that is, in the number of neutrons in the nucleus, for example hydrogen (no neutrons) and tritium (two neutrons).

62.   The correct answer is (A).

Carbon-12 (ordinary carbon) has 6 electrons, 6 protons, and 6 neutrons. Carbon-14 is an isotope of carbon and differs only in mass (i.e., neutron number). Hence, carbon-14 has 2 extra neutrons when compared to natural carbon. In summary, carbon-12 has 6 electrons, 6 protons, and 6 neutrons; carbon-14 has 6 electrons, 6 protons, and 6 neutrons.

63.   The correct answer is (B).

Gamma-ray decay is associated primarily with the emission of electromagnetic radiation, that is, photons. The internal rearrangement of the atom is responsible for gamma-ray emission, and there are no changes in the nuclear mass (i.e., the number of protons and neutrons) of the atom. Alpha decay is associated with a decrease of 4 units of atomic weight.

64.   The correct answer is (C).

The angstrom ($A°$) is 1×10^{-10} m., or 1×10^{-8} cm., the average radius of an atom.

65.   The correct answer is (D).

The prefix *pyro-* indicates loss of water. In this example, a molecule of water is lost from two molecules of orthophosphoric acid to form pyrophosphoric acid. The prefixes *hypo-* and *per-* refer, respectively, to the lowest and highest oxidation states. The prefix for the highest hydrated form is *ortho-*.

66.   The correct answer is (A).

Lead exists in the divalent (+2) and tetravalent (+4) oxidation states, where it is called the plumbus and plumbic ion, respectively. Copper also exists in two oxidation states, monovalent (+1) and divalent (+2).

67.   The correct answer is (B).

The alkaline-earth metals comprise group IIA of the periodic table. Phosphorus is not one of the elements in this group. Gypsum and plaster of paris are sulfate salts of calcium, the most abundant and useful element of group IIA. Plaster of paris is used to make plaster and surgical casts.

68.   The correct answer is (C).

Hydrogen sulfide gas not only smells obnoxious to the user, but it is also extremely toxic. It is a colorless gas, denser than air, and somewhat soluble in water; hence, the preparation and use of this gas should be carefully monitored.

69. The correct answer is (D).

CH$_3$COOH follows the general formula RCOOH, which represents an organic acid. This particular organic acid is acetic acid, commonly called vinegar. Aqua fortis is the common name for nitric acid. Aqua regia is a mixture of nitric and hydrochloric acids, while muriatic acid is commercially produced hydrochloric acid.

70. The correct answer is (D).

Baking soda is sodium bicarbonate, NaHCO$_3$. Sodium carbonate (Na$_2$CO$_3$) is washing soda and is used as a water softener. Na$_2$B$_4$O$_7$ is borax, while magnesium sulfate (MgSO$_4$) is known as Epsom salts.

71. The correct answer is (C).

HOCl is hypochlorous acid, formed from the initial reaction of chlorine gas and water. Most bleaching agents (e.g., Clorox) act by the release of hypochlorous acid into solution. Chloroform is an organic solvent (CHCl$_3$). Brine is the form of sodium chloride found in combination with sea water, while tincture of iodine is an alcoholic preparation containing iodine.

72. The correct answer is (B).

Alkenes have double bonds. This double bond is made up of one pi bond and one sigma bond. In organic chemistry there are no alpha bonds, but there are alpha-designated carbon atoms.

73. The correct answer is (A).

RCONH$_2$ are amides, the simplest member being formamide (HCONH$_2$). Acid anhydrides have the general formula (RCO)$_2$O, amines are generally RNH$_2$, while azides have the general formula RCON$_3$.

74. The correct answer is (C).

An enzyme usually has the suffix *-ase*, sugar usually ends in *-ose*, while a carboxyl group would end in *-ate*.

75. The correct answer is (A).

A tertiary (3°) alcohol has all of its alcohol carbon hydrogens substituted for other organic substituents; a secondary (2°) alcohol has only one hydrogen attached to the alcohol carbon; and a primary (1°) alcohol has only two hydrogens attached to the alcohol carbon. CH$_3$OH is methanol, which has only hydrogen attached to the alcohol carbon.

76. The correct answer is (B).

Vinyl usually refers to the CH$_2$ = CH radical. Thus, methyl vinyl ketone is CH$_3$COCH = CH$_2$. Ethyl vinyl ketone is CH$_3$CH$_2$COCH = CH$_2$. Butyric acid is CH$_3$CH$_2$CH$_2$COOH, whereas CH$_3$OCH$_2$CH = CH$_2$ is methyl allyl ether.

77. The correct answer is (D).

An organic acid is usually identified by the longest hydrocarbon chain, with the carboxyl carbon as carbon number 1. Changing the suffix from *-ane* to *-ol* would make it an alcohol and not an acid.

78.   The correct answer is (D).

$CH_3(CH_2)_8CH_3$ has ten carbon atoms; hence, it is called decane. Nonane has nine carbon atoms, while octane has only eight. Undecane is $C_{11}H_{24}$, and there are thus eleven carbon atoms in this saturated hydrocarbon.

79.   The correct answer is (C).

Atoms in double- or triple-bonded systems are rigid and not free to rotate around these bonds. Furthermore, ring systems have an aromatic character, and the atoms in these systems are also not free to rotate around their bonds. Only atoms connected by single bonds rotate around their sigma bonds.

80.   The correct answer is (B).

The carbonium ions, by definition, are atoms that contain a carbon atom with only six electrons. They are classified as primary, secondary, and tertiary ions, as in the classification of the organic alcohols. Since the stability of a carbonium ion is greatly increased by charge dispersal, a tertiary carbonium ion, which has three alkyl groups, is more stable than a secondary carbonium ion, which has two alkyl groups. The more stable the carbonium ion, the more easily it is formed.

81.   The correct answer is (D).

Benzene is a planar molecule; that is, all its atoms lie in the same plane. There are pi electron clouds above and below the plane of the ring, making it a rigid molecule with the formula C_6H_6. Each carbon atom lies at an angle of a regular six-sided figure, or hexagon. The bond angle is therefore 120°.

82.   The correct answer is (C).

Aldehyde and ketones have the carbonyl (—C = 0) functional group. The carbonyl carbon is joined to three other atoms by sigma bonds; there is also an overlap of a pi bond. The carbon hybridization orbitals are sp^2, and the molecule is planar, with bond angles of 120°.

83.   The correct answer is (B).

With regard to chemical reactivity and nucleophilic displacement, nucleophilic substitution occurs more readily at an acyl carbon (i.e., —RCO) than at a saturated carbon. Hence, a compound having a carbonyl group would be more prone to undergo nucleophilic substitution, for example, amides would be more prone than amines, acid chlorides more than alkyl chlorides, and esters more than ethers.

84.   The correct answer is (A).

Glycols are polyalcohols, usually containing two hydroxyl groups. These are saturated compounds, the simplest being ethylene glycol, CH_2OHCH_2OH. The suffix *-ol* should remind you that we are dealing with alcohols.

85.   The correct answer is (B).

The Grignard reagent is unique owing to its high reactivity. Its general formula is RMgX, and it is formed by reacting an alkyl halide with metallic magnesium in ether. The carbon-magnesium bond is highly polar but distinctly covalent (i.e., sharing of electrons); however, the magnesium-halogen bond is ionic in character.

86. The correct answer is (C).

Organic molecules are such that reactants must be optically active in order for the products to be optically active. The converse, that is, the relation between inactive reactants and inactive products, is also correct. However, the products of optically active reactants may not show such activity, and this is due to racemic modification of the isomers.

87. The correct answer is (D).

CH_4 is methane, and $—CH_3$ is the methyl radical of this alkane. CH_2 or methylene exists as a discrete molecule and is highly reactive. Methanol is formaldehyde, the former being the International Union of Pure and Applied Chemistry (IUPAC) nomenclature and the latter being the common name. Mesyl is the shortened form of the methyl sulfonyl radical and deals with sulfonic acid chemistry.

88. The correct answer is (D).

The Diels-Alder reaction is important because the end product of the reactants, a diene and a dienophile, is a six-membered ring. The diene usually possesses electron-releasing groups, while the dienophile (an $\alpha\beta$-unsaturated carbonyl compound) is associated with electron-withdrawing functional groups. Note that the Diels-Alder reaction is a reaction between a conjugated diene and an α-unsaturated carbonyl compound.

89. The correct answer is (A).

Disaccharides, on hydrolysis, yield two monosaccharides. Sucrose (cane sugar) will yield glucose and fructose. Maltose (malt sugar) will yield two molecules of glucose, while lactose (milk sugar) will yield glucose and galactose. Amylose is a water-soluble fraction of starch, a polysaccharide.

90. The correct answer is (C).

Amino acids have the general formula $RCHNH_2COOH$. The amino acid with the simplest structure is NH_2CH_2COOH, or glycine. Tyrosine is an aromatic amino acid, whereas arginine is a basic amino acid. Methionine is an amino acid containing an atom of sulfur.

91. The correct answer is (B).

Aryl halides are compounds in which the halogens are attached directly to the aromatic ring, for example, bromobenzene (C_6H_5Br). Alkyl halides are not only the saturated form of the halogen-containing compounds, for they also compose the substituted alkyl group, for example, vinyl chloride.

92. The correct answer is (D).

The catalytic addition of oxygen to ethylene ($CH_2 = CH_2$) results in the formation of ethylene oxide, which has the structure:

$$CH_2 \overset{\textstyle\diagdown\quad\diagup}{\underset{\textstyle O}{\rule{0pt}{0pt}}} CH_2$$

Ethylene oxide is therefore an epoxide, whereas ethylene is an alkene.

93.   The correct answer is (C).

Amines have the general formula RNH_2. Primary amines have the formula RNH_2, secondary amines have the formula R_2NH, and tertiary amines have the formula R_3N. RNH is an amine radical and lacks either an R group or a hydrogen atom.

94.   The correct answer is (C).

One hundred percent alcohol (or 200 proof alcohol) is absolute alcohol or water-free alcohol. Methanol is synonymous with wood alcohol. Absolute alcohol absorbs various amounts of water from the atmosphere and must be stored accordingly.

95.   The correct answer is (A).

The simplest member of the fused-ring hydrocarbon family is naphthalene, which has two benzene rings. Anthracene has three fused benzene rings, just like phenanthrene.

96.   The correct answer is (B).

CH_3OH is the formula for an organic alcohol commonly known as methanol. Menthone is a long-chained organic compound (i.e., a terpene) with a keto group, whereas mesitol is trimethyl phenol, an alkyl-substituted aryl alcohol. Menthol is a cyclic alcohol derived from mint oils.

97.   The correct answer is (C).

Tollen's reagent contains $[Ag(NH_3)_2]^+$, the silver ammonium ion. Oxidation of an aldehyde to an acid is accompanied by the formation of a silver mirror. The latter is the result of the reduction of the soluble silver ion to yield free silver metal.

98.   The correct answer is (D).

Ammonia has the formula NH_3. Nitrogen uses four sp^3 orbitals in forming this molecule; they are directed toward the corners of a regular tetrahedron, with one orbital containing a pair of electrons. The other three each contain a single electron.

99.   The correct answer is (B).

By converting an organic acid to an acid chloride, we can produce a substance from which we can form esters and amides. Acid chlorides are much more reactive than their original acid and are therefore quite useful. Because of their reactivity, thionyl chloride and the chlorides of phosphorus are commonly employed in the preparation of acid chlorides. Note that these compounds have sulfur or phosphorus as the inorganic element. Ethyl chloride is a substituted halogenated hydrocarbon and plays no role in the preparation of such acid chlorides.

100.   The correct answer is (A).

All monosaccharides are reducing sugars, that is, they reduce Tollen's or Fehling's reagent. These monosaccharides can be aldo or keto sugars. Glucose is a monosaccharide and hence a reducing sugar. Most disaccharides are reducing sugars as well. Even though sucrose is a disaccharide, it does not reduce Tollen's or Fehling's solution.

Chapter 10: Reading Comprehension

This section is comprised of nine reading passages. Each of the passages is either short (200-600 words) or long (700-950 words), and is followed by a set of questions that directly relate to the passage. There are usually 4-6 questions with short passages and 8-12 questions for long passages. The passages selected for the actual PCAT come from different content areas, including biology, chemistry, and the physical sciences. The actual test contains both long and short passages with a total of five or six passages.

KEY POINTS TO REMEMBER

1. Reading comprehension is based on your reading skills, including understanding new words, developing speed and rhythm in your reading style, and scanning passages quickly and correlating information.

2. The PCAT tests your ability to read, organize, and analyze information.

3. Because the information explosion is doubling the amount of available information every two years, you will need to be able to read and comprehend a significant amount of literature in a short time.

4. New information refers to information that you have not yet seen and information that you have seen at a glance. For instance, in the *Wall Street Journal*, articles are briefly recapped on the front page. It is important to be able to scan these recaps for recognition of new information.

5. Reading ability depends on the complexity and difficulty of the reading.

6. You must be able to concentrate on reading passages without trying to memorize information as you read.

7. Improve your vocabulary daily. Working on crossword puzzles and keeping a log or diary of new words are two ways to increase vocabulary.

8. The level of a reading passage is dependent upon the topic as well as the vocabulary used in the passage. Increasing your vocabulary will enhance your reading comprehension as well as your verbal ability.

9. Reason as you read! If a passage has long complex sentences, break them down into manageable components that you can absorb and analyze. Understanding short phrases will assist you in reading and comprehending complex passages.

10. There are several sources of new information that you should begin reading routinely. You do not have to buy these publications; you can read them in the library or your local bookstore. These include, but are not limited to, the following:

American Journal of Hospital Pharmacy

American Journal of Managed Care

American Pharmacy

Journal of the American Medical Association

Nature

PharmacoEconomics

Science

The New England Journal of Medicine

The Wall Street Journal

Time

USA Today

Local newspapers

11. Practice reading passages from some of the above sources. For this exercise, use the following techniques:

- Take approximately 30–45 seconds to scan the passage.

- Find the primary topic covered in the passage.

- Read the questions to get concepts, not the answer choices.

- Go back and read the passage (2–5 minutes) and develop correlations between the questions and the content of the passage. You may want to underline concepts in the passage that relate to the questions.

- Mark your answers on the answer sheet.

Remember: you can go back to the passage whenever you need to.

12. Do not read in haste!

13. Read and focus on the topic area as well as on the questions. Do NOT answer the questions based on your knowledge, but rather on the information provided in the passage. While your knowledge may be absolutely correct, the passage may focus on a different approach to the topic.

14. You may not agree with the statements in the passage, but keep in mind that you are reading to comprehend what appears in the passage.

Answer Sheet

Chapter 10: Reading Comprehension

1. Ⓐ Ⓑ Ⓒ Ⓓ   10. Ⓐ Ⓑ Ⓒ Ⓓ   19. Ⓐ Ⓑ Ⓒ Ⓓ   28. Ⓐ Ⓑ Ⓒ Ⓓ   37. Ⓐ Ⓑ Ⓒ Ⓓ

2. Ⓐ Ⓑ Ⓒ Ⓓ   11. Ⓐ Ⓑ Ⓒ Ⓓ   20. Ⓐ Ⓑ Ⓒ Ⓓ   29. Ⓐ Ⓑ Ⓒ Ⓓ   38. Ⓐ Ⓑ Ⓒ Ⓓ

3. Ⓐ Ⓑ Ⓒ Ⓓ   12. Ⓐ Ⓑ Ⓒ Ⓓ   21. Ⓐ Ⓑ Ⓒ Ⓓ   30. Ⓐ Ⓑ Ⓒ Ⓓ   39. Ⓐ Ⓑ Ⓒ Ⓓ

4. Ⓐ Ⓑ Ⓒ Ⓓ   13. Ⓐ Ⓑ Ⓒ Ⓓ   22. Ⓐ Ⓑ Ⓒ Ⓓ   31. Ⓐ Ⓑ Ⓒ Ⓓ   40. Ⓐ Ⓑ Ⓒ Ⓓ

5. Ⓐ Ⓑ Ⓒ Ⓓ   14. Ⓐ Ⓑ Ⓒ Ⓓ   23. Ⓐ Ⓑ Ⓒ Ⓓ   32. Ⓐ Ⓑ Ⓒ Ⓓ   41. Ⓐ Ⓑ Ⓒ Ⓓ

6. Ⓐ Ⓑ Ⓒ Ⓓ   15. Ⓐ Ⓑ Ⓒ Ⓓ   24. Ⓐ Ⓑ Ⓒ Ⓓ   33. Ⓐ Ⓑ Ⓒ Ⓓ   42. Ⓐ Ⓑ Ⓒ Ⓓ

7. Ⓐ Ⓑ Ⓒ Ⓓ   16. Ⓐ Ⓑ Ⓒ Ⓓ   25. Ⓐ Ⓑ Ⓒ Ⓓ   34. Ⓐ Ⓑ Ⓒ Ⓓ   43. Ⓐ Ⓑ Ⓒ Ⓓ

8. Ⓐ Ⓑ Ⓒ Ⓓ   17. Ⓐ Ⓑ Ⓒ Ⓓ   26. Ⓐ Ⓑ Ⓒ Ⓓ   35. Ⓐ Ⓑ Ⓒ Ⓓ   44. Ⓐ Ⓑ Ⓒ Ⓓ

9. Ⓐ Ⓑ Ⓒ Ⓓ   18. Ⓐ Ⓑ Ⓒ Ⓓ   27. Ⓐ Ⓑ Ⓒ Ⓓ   36. Ⓐ Ⓑ Ⓒ Ⓓ   45. Ⓐ Ⓑ Ⓒ Ⓓ

Tear Here

Reading Comprehension Practice Questions

45 QUESTIONS—45 MINUTES

Directions: Read each of the following passages and choose the best answer to the questions that follow each passage.

Questions 1–5 are based on the following passage.

Line Before the intravenous administration of a medication, it is essential to check the medication, dose, fluid in which the drug is to be given, and time of administration against the patient's chart.
(5) After this, all the necessary equipment, such as an alcohol or iodophor sponge, a needle, an intravenous board, tape, and the intravenous solution or admixture, should be assembled. The patient should then be identified by his armband
(10) and the procedure explained to the patient to alleviate any apprehension. Venipuncture can then be performed using a needle or catheter that should be checked after insertion to ensure that it is properly placed in the vein and ad-
(15) equately secured to the patient's arm. The patient should be advised not to disturb the venipuncture site. Because the rate of flow of the solution can be affected by numerous variables (gravity, solution viscosity, temperature, and pos-
(20) sibly defective equipment), it should be checked every hour or so, depending on hospital policy. When the rate of flow is critical, such as in pediatric patients or in parenteral nutrition, an infusion pump may be needed to ensure the proper
(25) flow of solution into the patient.

1. Which of the following items is NOT part of the necessary equipment for administering an intravenous medication?
   (A) Alcohol sponge or swab
   (B) Needle
   (C) Intravenous solution
   (D) Intramuscular solution

2. Which of the following is a variable that affects the rate of flow of medication?
   (A) Solution color
   (B) Solution viscosity
   (C) Solution smell
   (D) Solution particle size

3. On what kinds of patients should an infusion pump be used?
   (A) Pediatric patients
   (B) Adult patients
   (C) Geriatric patients
   (D) Comatose patients

4. Before administering an intravenous solution one must check the
   (A) time.
   (B) medication against the chart.
   (C) day.
   (D) dose of the intramuscular drug.

5. After administering an intravenous solution, the rate of flow should be checked
   (A) every hour.
   (B) every half hour.
   (C) periodically.
   (D) per the time specified by hospital policy.

Questions 6–10 are based on the following passage.

Line Adrenergic agents, commonly found in appetite suppressants, bronchodilators, central nervous system stimulants, and vasoconstrictors, produce slight pupillary dilation. They have not been
(5) observed to produce any adverse effects in open-angle glaucoma, and the incidence of deleterious effects on angle closure glaucoma after systemic administration has been extremely low. Adrenergic agents such as epinephrine and phe-
(10) nylephrine have been used ocularly to treat open-angle glaucoma. It is important to note, however, that these agents will elevate the intraocular pressure by narrowing the anterior chamber angle when instilled into eyes of angle
(15) closure patients.

General anesthetics producing parasympathetic and sympathetic imbalance may cause pupillary block. To prevent this complication, topical pilocarpine at 1% may be instilled into the
(20) eye 1 hour prior to anesthesia.

6. Adrenergic agents are commonly found in all of the following EXCEPT

   (A) bronchodilators.

   (B) bronchoconstrictors.

   (C) vasoconstrictors.

   (D) appetite suppressants.

7. General anesthetics that produce parasympathetic and sympathetic imbalance may cause pupillary

   (A) constriction.

   (B) dilation.

   (C) block.

   (D) stimulation.

8. Adrenergic agents may cause _____ in intraocular pressure.

   (A) a decrease

   (B) an increase

   (C) a slight change

   (D) no change

9. Which adrenergic agents have been used to treat open-angle glaucoma?

   (A) Epinephrine and ACTH

   (B) Epinephrine and propranolol

   (C) Epinephrine and phenylephrine

   (D) Epinephrine and droperidol

10. Pilocarpine administered _____ hour(s) before anesthesia can prevent the pupillary block caused by anesthetics.

   (A) 4

   (B) 2

   (C) $1\frac{1}{2}$

   (D) 1

Questions 11–15 are based on the following passage.

Line There are numerous methods of administering diphenylhydantoin; however, the regimen must be prescribed individually for each patient because of the many variables that influence the
(5) absorption, distribution, metabolism, and excretion of diphenylhydantoin. Ventricular tachycardia usually requires intravenous therapy. There appears to be no indication in this situation for intramuscular injections, because the drug is
(10) slowly and erratically absorbed from the site, besides being very painful. Diphenylhydantoin plasma levels after intramuscular injection may be 25-50% lower than after equivalent oral doses. Doses of 50-100 mg. of diphenylhydan-
(15) toin, up to a maximum of 1.0 g., may be admin-

istered intravenously every 5 minutes, producing only a mild decrease (10–30 mmHg) in systolic blood pressure. Single intravenous doses of 300 mg. or more produce a more marked (20) hypotension (20–45 mmHg) and also lead to subtherapeutic diphenylhydantoin plasma levels within 20–40 minutes. Generally, cardiovascular complications can be avoided with an infusion rate of 20–50 mg./min.

11. Treatment of ventricular tachycardia with diphenylhydantoin usually requires

   (A) sublingual therapy.

   (B) intramuscular therapy.

   (C) intravenous therapy.

   (D) subcutaneous therapy.

12. The dose of diphenylhydantoin that may be given intravenously is

   (A) 50–70 mg.

   (B) 50–80 mg.

   (C) 50–100 mg.

   (D) 50–120 mg.

13. With which infusion rate can you avoid cardiovascular complications?

   (A) 20–50 mg./min.

   (B) 20–40 mg./min.

   (C) 20–30 mg./min.

   (D) 10–50 mg./min.

14. At what dose would you expect to see a marked hypotensive effect from diphenylhydantoin?

   (A) 100 mg.

   (B) 200 mg.

   (C) 250 mg.

   (D) 300 mg.

15. Which of the following is a reason for NOT administering diphenylhydantoin intramuscularly?

   (A) The procedure is too expensive.

   (B) The drug is erratically absorbed at the site.

   (C) The drug is not absorbed at the site.

   (D) The drug is too unstable.

Questions 16–20 are based on the following passage.

Line In open-angle glaucoma a physical blockage occurs within the trabecular meshwork that retards elimination of aqueous humor. The obstruction is presumed to be located between the tra-
(5) becular sheet and the episcleral veins, into which the aqueous humor ultimately flows. The impairment of aqueous drainage elevates the intraocular pressure (IOP) to 25–35 mmHg (normal, 10–20 mmHg), indicating that the obstruction is
(10) usually partial. This increase in IOP is sufficient to cause progressive cupping of the optic disk and eventual visual field defects. As the trabecular spaces become more involved, detachment of the cornea and formation of bullae may de-
(15) velop. In addition, scotomata (blind spots) may develop. Since visual acuity remains largely unaffected until late in the disease, presence of scotomata must be regarded as a major indication for the institution of medical therapy.

16. Open-angle glaucoma is caused by

(A) physical blockage.

(B) genetics.

(C) physical drainage.

(D) infection.

17. Normal IOP has a range of

(A) 10-15 mmHg.

(B) 10-25 mmHg.

(C) 10-20 mmHg.

(D) 10-30 mmHg.

18. Increases in IOP may cause all of the following EXCEPT

(A) progressive cupping of the optic disk.

(B) visual field defects (over time).

(C) immediate changes in visual field.

(D) development of scotomas.

19. Impairment of aqueous drainage elevates the IOP to

(A) 25–30 mmHg.

(B) 25–35 mmHg.

(C) 25–40 mmHg.

(D) 25–45 mmHg.

20. The obstruction in open-angle glaucoma is presumed to be located between the

(A) cornea and the iris.

(B) trabecular sheet and the episcleral veins.

(C) trabecular sheet and the cornea.

(D) episcleral veins and the cornea.

Questions 21–25 are based on the following passage.

Line An unusual reaction to quinidine is syncope. Besides loss of consciousness, these syncopal attacks involve pallor, muscular twitching, and sometimes seizures. When an EKG is obtained
(5) during an attack, the pattern indicates ventricular tachyarrhythmia that apparently critically decreases cerebral perfusion, causing loss of consciousness. The attacks usually terminate spontaneously, but the rare cases of sudden death
(10) attributed to quinidine are thought to be secondary to ventricular arrhythmia. On the other hand, this condition is often observed in patients with coronary artery disease, where sudden death has been reported to occur as a result of
(15) the primary cardiac pathological condition rather than from the drug itself. Syncope may occur at low doses (e.g., 0.8 g./day) and without evidence of allergic reactions. An adverse dose-related effect is hypotension, which may
(20) occur by alpha-adrenergic receptor blockade or by a direct negative inotropic effect on the heart.

21. Which of the following is NOT associated with syncopal attacks?

(A) Pallor

(B) Muscular twitching

(C) Loss of consciousness

(D) Itching

22. An adverse dose-related effect of quinidine is

(A) hypertension.

(B) hypotension.

(C) an inotropic effect.

(D) diabetes.

23. When an EKG is obtained during an attack, the pattern indicates

(A) arrhythmia.

(B) ventricular tachyarrhythmia.

(C) ventricular flutter.

(D) atrial tachyarrhythmia.

24. An unusual reaction to quinidine is

(A) ataxia.

(B) pallor.

(C) syncope.

(D) hypotension.

25. Syncope may occur at

(A) high doses of quinidine.

(B) moderate doses of quinidine.

(C) low doses of quinidine.

(D) very high doses of quinidine.

Questions 26–30 are based on the following passage.

Line Many reports have indicated that the tricyclic antidepressants, especially imipramine, may be of benefit in the treatment of MBD in children. However, although most studies have indicated
(5) their superiority over placebos, they are still not as effective as the psychostimulants. Further drawbacks associated with their use include the development of tolerance in some children and numerous deleterious side effects. Side effects
(10) may be somewhat limited by the maximum daily dose approved by the FDA (5 mg./kg. per day), but the patient must be regularly examined for autonomic effects, weight loss, gastrointestinal irritation, fine tremors, hyperirritability, and
(15) mood alterations. In addition, the patient should be monitored for more severe effects on the central nervous system, for example, seizures, and the cardiovascular system, but these can usually be avoided if the practitioner adheres to

(20) FDA recommendations. Although the tricyclic antidepressants are helpful in the treatment of MBD in children, their use at this point is experimental and must be accompanied by certain precautions.

26. Which of the following tricyclic antidepressants has been reported to be effective with MBD?

(A) Desipramine

(B) Imipramine

(C) Amitriptyline

(D) Doxepin

27. The maximum daily dose of tricyclic antipressants approved by the FDA is

(A) 5 mg./kg. per day.

(B) 10 mg./kg. per day.

(C) 15 mg./kg. per day.

(D) 20 mg./kg. per day.

28. While the tricyclic antidepressants are superior to placebos, they are still not as effective as

(A) hypnotics.

(B) sedatives.

(C) psychostimulants.

(D) stimulants.

29. The patient must be monitored for more severe side effects on the central nervous system such as

(A) dizziness.

(B) seizures.

(C) headaches.

(D) blindness.

30. Another drawback associated with the use of the tricyclics is

(A) the development of addiction.

(B) sedation.

(C) the development of physical addiction.

(D) the development of tolerance.

Questions 31–35 are based on the following passage.

Line The primary agents in the treatment of MBD are the centrally acting sympathomimetics, for example, methylphenidate, dextroamphetamine, and magnesium pemoline. This therapeutic ap-
(5) proach was first used in 1937, but actual definition and characterization of this indication in pediatric psychopharmacology did not become popular until the late 1960s. Dextroamphetamine was initially used in 1937 and continued
(10) to be the agent of choice until the late 1960s, when methylphenidate usage increased in association with reports of a lower incidence of side effects with the latter drug. It would appear that these reports of the greater safety of meth-
(15) ylphenidate therapy are of questionable clinical significance. Studies attesting to the greater clinical efficacy of methylphenidate over dextroamphetamine have also been carried out by some authorities who prefer the use of the former
(20) drug, while proponents of dextroamphetamine indicate that, in their hands, it has comparable clinical efficacy at a lower cost.

31. The agent of choice in the treatment of MBD until the late 1960s was

(A) amitriptyline.

(B) dextroamphetamine.

(C) methylphenidate.

(D) magnesium pemoline.

32. Which of the following involves the lowest cost in the treatment of MBD?

(A) Dextroamphetamine

(B) Methylphenidate

(C) Amitriptyline

(D) None of the above

33. Which of the following is NOT a primary agent in the treatment of MBD?

(A) Methylphenidate

(B) Magnesium pemoline

(C) Dextroamphetamine

(D) Chlorpromazine

34. Methylphenidate use increased in the late 1960s due to reports of its

(A) lower cost.

(B) decreased risk of addiction.

(C) lower incidence of side effects.

(D) shorter half-life.

35. The reports of the greater safety of methylphenidate therapy are

(A) conclusive.

(B) still in progress.

(C) of questionable significance.

(D) accepted by all.

Questions 36–40 are based on the following passage.

Line Procainamide may be considered as an alternative to quinidine in the treatment and prophylaxis of atrial fibrillation. Most patients absorb 75-95% of an oral dose; however, Koch-Weser
(5) estimated that 10% of subjects may absorb 50% or less. The uncertainty concerning the dose absorbed and the lag time for stomach emptying into the small bowel, where the drug is

finally absorbed, force the parenteral adminis-
(10) tration of procainamide in emergencies.
Procainamide may be given intravenously at a
rate of 25–50 mg./min. Giardina et al. have intravenously administered 100 mg., up to a maximum of 1 g., every 5 minutes to treat ventricu-
(15) lar arrhythmia. This method will produce a mini-
mally effective serum concentration in 15 minutes. Therapy never had to be interrupted because of hypotension or conduction distur-
bances; however, the investigators had excluded
(20) myocardial infarction patients, who are most sus-
ceptible to these adverse reactions, from their
population.

---

36. Which of the following drugs may be considered as an alternative to quinidine?

(A) Propranolol

(B) Procainamide

(C) Digoxin

(D) Aspirin

---

37. The dosage used by Giardina et al. to treat ventricular arrhythmias was

(A) 100 mg. intravenously every 5 minutes.

(B) 100 mg. intramuscularly every 5 minutes.

(C) 200 mg. intravenously every 5 minutes.

(D) 200 mg. intramuscularly every 5 minutes.

---

38. The normal rate of intravenous administration of procainamide is

(A) 25–100 mg./min.

(B) 25–75 mg./min.

(C) 25–125 mg./min.

(D) 25–50 mg./min.

39. Most patients absorb what percentage of an oral dose of procainamide?

(A) 65–75%

(B) 65–95%

(C) 75–95%

(D) 55–75%

40. Koch-Weser estimates that 10% of the patients will absorb

(A) 50% or less.

(B) 60% or less.

(C) 70% or less.

(D) 80% or less.

Questions 41–45 are based on the following passage.

Line Corticosteroid-induced glaucoma is well docu-
mented. This form of glaucoma is usually painless and involves no ocular findings or visual field
defects. The blockage produced probably occurs
(5) in the trabecular meshwork, severely decreasing the outflow of aqueous humor. Systemically
or topically administered corticosteroids further
hinder outflow, causing a corresponding increase in intraocular pressure. After topical
(10) therapy, a glaucomatous change occurs in the
eye instilled with the drug. This ocular hypertensive effect is usually fully reversible within
one month after discontinuation of steroid
therapy. The increase in intraocular pressure is
(15) approximately 10 mmHg for patients with
preglaucomatous anterior chambers, and 5
mmHg for normal persons. In some cases, irreversible eye damage occurs if ocular tension
persists for one to two months or longer. In ad-
(20) dition, cupping of the optic disk and visual field
defects may develop a few months after topical
administration of corticosteroids has begun. Patients undergoing chronic topical steroid
therapy should therefore have a tonometric ex-
(25) amination every two months.

41. The increase in intraocular pressure is approximately at what level for patients with preglaucomatous anterior chambers?

    (A) 5 mmHg

    (B) 10 mmHg

    (C) 15 mmHg

    (D) 20 mmHg

42. The ocular hypertensive effect caused by corticosteroids is usually

    (A) irreversible.

    (B) fully reversible.

    (C) not seen.

    (D) partially reversible.

43. Irreversible eye damage may occur if ocular hypertension persists for

    (A) two to four months.

    (B) one to two months.

    (C) one to four months.

    (D) two to six months.

44. Corticosteroid-induced glaucoma usually does not involve any of the following symptoms EXCEPT

    (A) pain.

    (B) physical findings in the eye.

    (C) cupping of the optic disk.

    (D) night blindness.

45. Patients undergoing chronic topical corticosteroid therapy should have a tonometric every

    (A) month.

    (B) 2 months.

    (C) 3 months.

    (D) 4 months.

ANSWER KEY

Reading Comprehension				
1. D	10. D	19. B	28. C	37. A
2. B	11. C	20. B	29. B	38. D
3. A	12. C	21. D	30. D	39. C
4. B	13. A	22. B	31. B	40. A
5. D	14. D	23. B	32. A	41. B
6. B	15. B	24. C	33. D	42. B
7. C	16. A	25. C	34. C	43. B
8. B	17. C	26. B	35. C	44. C
9. C	18. C	27. A	36. B	45. B

EXPLANATORY ANSWERS

1. **The correct answer is (D).**

   The answer to this question is found in **line 7** of the paragraph. An intramuscular solution is given intramuscularly rather than intravenously.

2. **The correct answer is (B).**

   The answer is found in **lines 19 and 20** of the paragraph. There are several variables, including the answer, that affect the rate of flow of medication: gravity, temperature, and possibly the equipment itself.

3. **The correct answer is (A).**

   The answer is found in **lines 22–25**: "When the rate of flow is critical, such as in pediatric patients or in parenteral nutrition, an infusion pump may be needed to ensure the proper flow of solution into the patient."

4. **The correct answer is (B).**

   The answer is found in **lines 1–4** of the paragraph: "Before the intravenous administration of a medication, it is essential to check the medication, the dose, fluid in which the drug is to be given, and time of administration against the patient's chart."

5. **The correct answer is (D).**

   The answer is found in **lines 20–21** of the paragraph: "…it should be checked every hour or so, depending on hospital policy."

6. **The correct answer is (B).**

   The answer is found in **lines 1–3** of the paragraph. Bronchoconstrictors do not appear in the list of items in which adrenergic agents are commonly found.

7. **The correct answer is (C).**

   The answer is found in **lines 16–18** of the paragraph: "General anesthetics producing parasympathetic and sympathetic imbalance may cause pupillary block."

8. **The correct answer is (B).**

   The answer is found in **lines 11–12** of the paragraph: "It is important to note, however, that these agents will elevate the intraocular pressure by narrowing the anterior chamber angle when instilled into eyes of angle closure patients."

9. **The correct answer is (C).**

   The answer is found in **lines 9–11** of the paragraph: "Adrenergic agents such as epinephrine and phenylephrine have been used ocularly to treat open-angle glaucoma."

10. **The correct answer is (D).**

    The answer is found in **lines 18–20** of the paragraph: "To prevent this complication, topical pilocarpine at 1% may be instilled into the eye 1 hour prior to anesthesia."

11. **The correct answer is (C).**

    The answer is found in **lines 6 and 7** of the paragraph: "Ventricular tachycardia usually requires intravenous therapy."

12. **The correct answer is (C).**

    The answer is found in **lines 14–16** of the paragraph: "Doses of 50-100 mg. of diphenylhydantoin, up to a maximum of 1.0 g., may be administered intravenously every 5 minutes."

13. **The correct answer is (A).**

The answer is found in **lines 22 and 23** of the paragraph: "Generally, cardiovascular complications can be avoided with an infusion rate of 20–50 mg./min."

14. **The correct answer is (D).**

The answer is found in **lines 18–21** of the paragraph: "Single intravenous doses of 300 mg. or more produce a more marked hypotension (20–45 mmHg) and also lead to subtherapeutic diphenylhydantoin plasma levels."

15. **The correct answer is (B).**

The answer is found in **lines 7–11** of the paragraph: "There appears to be no indication in this situation for intramuscular injections, because the drug is slowly and erratically absorbed from the site, besides being very painful."

16. **The correct answer is (A).**

The answer is found in **lines 1–3** of the paragraph: "In open-angle glaucoma a physical blockage occurs within the trabecular meshwork that retards elimination."

17. **The correct answer is (C).**

The answer is found in **lines 8–9** of the paragraph. The normal intraocular pressure is l0–20 mmHg.

18. **The correct answer is (C).**

The answer is found in **lines 10–12** of the paragraph. Visual field effects occur eventually and only after the disease has been present for a period of time. The changes are not immediate.

19. **The correct answer is (B).**

The answer is found in **lines 6–8** of the paragraph: "The impairment of aqueous drainage elevates the intraocular pressure (IOP) to 25-35 mmHg."

20. **The correct answer is (B).**

The answer is found in **lines 3–5** of the paragraph: "The obstruction is presumed to be located between the trabecular sheet and the episcleral veins."

21. **The correct answer is (D).**

The answer is found in **lines 2–4** of the paragraph: "Besides loss of consciousness, these syncopal attacks involve pallor, muscular twitching, and sometimes seizures."

22. **The correct answer is (B).**

The answer is found in **lines 18–21** of the paragraph: "An adverse dose-related effect is hypotension, which may occur by alpha-adrenergic receptor blockade or by a direct negative inotropic effect on the heart."

23. **The correct answer is (B).**

The answer is found in **lines 4–6** of the paragraph: "When an EKG is obtained during an attack, the pattern indicates ventricular tachyarrhythmia."

24. **The correct answer is (C).**

The answer is found in **line 1** of the paragraph: "An unusual reaction to quinidine is syncope."

25. **The correct answer is (C).**

The answer is found in **lines 16–17** of the paragraph: "Syncope may occur at low doses (e.g., 0.8 g./day)."

26. **The correct answer is (B).**

The answer is found in **lines 1–3** of the paragraph: "Many reports have indicated that the tricyclic antidepressants, especially imipramine, may be of benefit in the treatment of MBD in children."

27. **The correct answer is (A).**

    The answer is found in **lines 10 and 11** of the paragraph: " . . . the maximum daily dose approved by the FDA (5 mg./kg. per day) . . ."

28. **The correct answer is (C).**

    The answer is found in **lines 4–6** of the paragraph: "However, although most studies have indicated their superiority over placebos, they are still not as effective as the psychostimulants."

29. **The correct answer is (B).**

    The answer is found in **lines 15–17** of the paragraph: "In addition, the patient should be monitored for more severe effects on the central nervous system, for example, seizures."

30. **The correct answer is (D).**

    The answer is found in **lines 6–9** of the paragraph: "Further drawbacks associated with their use include the development of tolerance in some children and numerous deleterious side effects."

31. **The correct answer is (B).**

    The answer is found in **lines 8–10** of the paragraph: "Dextroamphetamine was initially used in 1937 and continued to be the agent of choice until the late 1960s."

32. **The correct answer is (A).**

    The answer is found in **lines 20–22** of the paragraph: " . . . while proponents of dextroamphetamine indicate that, in their hands, it has comparable clinical efficacy at a lower cost."

33. **The correct answer is (D).**

    The answer is found in **lines 1–4** of the paragraph: "The primary agents in the treatment of MBD are the centrally acting sympathomimetics, for example, methylphenidate, dextroamphetamine, and magnesium pemoline."

34. **The correct answer is (C).**

    The answer is found in **lines 11–13** of the paragraph: "Methylphenidate usage increased in association with reports of a lower incidence of side effects with the latter drug."

35. **The correct answer is (C).**

    The answer is found in **lines 13–16** of the paragraph: "It would appear that these reports of the greater safety of methylphenidate therapy are of questionable clinical significance."

36. **The correct answer is (B).**

    The answer is found in **lines 1–2** of the paragraph: "Procainamide may be considered as an alternative to quinidine."

37. **The correct answer is (A).**

    The answer is found in **lines 12–15** of the paragraph: "Giardina et al. have intravenously administered 100 mg., up to a maximum of 1 g., every 5 minutes to treat ventricular arrhythmia."

38. **The correct answer is (D).**

    The answer is found in **lines 11–12** of the paragraph: "Procainamide may be given intravenously at a rate of 25-50 mg./min."

39. **The correct answer is (C).**

    The answer is found in **lines 3–4** of the paragraph: "Most patients absorb 75-95% of an oral dose."

40.   The correct answer is (A).

The answer is found in **lines 4–6** of the paragraph: "However, Koch-Weser estimated that 10% of subjects may absorb 50% or less."

41.   The correct answer is (B).

The answer is found in **lines 14–16** of the paragraph: "The increase in intraocular pressure is approximately 10 mmHg for patients with preglaucomatous anterior chambers."

42.   The correct answer is (B).

The answer is found in **lines 11–13** of the paragraph: "This ocular hypertensive effect is usually fully reversible within one month after discontinuation of steroid therapy."

43.   The correct answer is (B).

The answer is found in **lines 17–19** of the paragraph: "In some cases, irreversible eye damage occurs if ocular tension persists for one to two months or longer."

44.   The correct answer is (C).

The answer is found in **lines 2–4** of the paragraph: "This form of glaucoma is usually painless and involves no ocular findings or visual field defects."

45.   The correct answer is (B).

The answer is found in **lines 22–25** of the paragraph: "Patients undergoing chronic topical steroid therapy should therefore have a tonometric examination every two months."

PART IV

Practice PCAT Examination

Chapter 11: Practice Examination

INSTRUCTIONS

The following is a full-length PCAT practice examination that simulates the actual examination. Note that the order in which the sections are arranged and the number of questions in this practice examination may not be the same as the actual examination you take. Also note that the PCAT has an additional section that is experimental and does count toward your final score. This practice examination does not include the experimental section. An answer key and explanations follow the examination. Do not look at the answer section until you have completed the entire practice examination.

Answer Sheet

Reading Comprehension: 45 questions, #1–45

1. Ⓐ Ⓑ Ⓒ Ⓓ	10. Ⓐ Ⓑ Ⓒ Ⓓ	19. Ⓐ Ⓑ Ⓒ Ⓓ	28. Ⓐ Ⓑ Ⓒ Ⓓ	37. Ⓐ Ⓑ Ⓒ Ⓓ
2. Ⓐ Ⓑ Ⓒ Ⓓ	11. Ⓐ Ⓑ Ⓒ Ⓓ	20. Ⓐ Ⓑ Ⓒ Ⓓ	29. Ⓐ Ⓑ Ⓒ Ⓓ	38. Ⓐ Ⓑ Ⓒ Ⓓ
3. Ⓐ Ⓑ Ⓒ Ⓓ	12. Ⓐ Ⓑ Ⓒ Ⓓ	21. Ⓐ Ⓑ Ⓒ Ⓓ	30. Ⓐ Ⓑ Ⓒ Ⓓ	39. Ⓐ Ⓑ Ⓒ Ⓓ
4. Ⓐ Ⓑ Ⓒ Ⓓ	13. Ⓐ Ⓑ Ⓒ Ⓓ	22. Ⓐ Ⓑ Ⓒ Ⓓ	31. Ⓐ Ⓑ Ⓒ Ⓓ	40. Ⓐ Ⓑ Ⓒ Ⓓ
5. Ⓐ Ⓑ Ⓒ Ⓓ	14. Ⓐ Ⓑ Ⓒ Ⓓ	23. Ⓐ Ⓑ Ⓒ Ⓓ	32. Ⓐ Ⓑ Ⓒ Ⓓ	41. Ⓐ Ⓑ Ⓒ Ⓓ
6. Ⓐ Ⓑ Ⓒ Ⓓ	15. Ⓐ Ⓑ Ⓒ Ⓓ	24. Ⓐ Ⓑ Ⓒ Ⓓ	33. Ⓐ Ⓑ Ⓒ Ⓓ	42. Ⓐ Ⓑ Ⓒ Ⓓ
7. Ⓐ Ⓑ Ⓒ Ⓓ	16. Ⓐ Ⓑ Ⓒ Ⓓ	25. Ⓐ Ⓑ Ⓒ Ⓓ	34. Ⓐ Ⓑ Ⓒ Ⓓ	43. Ⓐ Ⓑ Ⓒ Ⓓ
8. Ⓐ Ⓑ Ⓒ Ⓓ	17. Ⓐ Ⓑ Ⓒ Ⓓ	26. Ⓐ Ⓑ Ⓒ Ⓓ	35. Ⓐ Ⓑ Ⓒ Ⓓ	44. Ⓐ Ⓑ Ⓒ Ⓓ
9. Ⓐ Ⓑ Ⓒ Ⓓ	18. Ⓐ Ⓑ Ⓒ Ⓓ	27. Ⓐ Ⓑ Ⓒ Ⓓ	36. Ⓐ Ⓑ Ⓒ Ⓓ	45. Ⓐ Ⓑ Ⓒ Ⓓ

Verbal Ability: 50 questions, #46–95

46. Ⓐ Ⓑ Ⓒ Ⓓ	56. Ⓐ Ⓑ Ⓒ Ⓓ	66. Ⓐ Ⓑ Ⓒ Ⓓ	76. Ⓐ Ⓑ Ⓒ Ⓓ	86. Ⓐ Ⓑ Ⓒ Ⓓ
47. Ⓐ Ⓑ Ⓒ Ⓓ	57. Ⓐ Ⓑ Ⓒ Ⓓ	67. Ⓐ Ⓑ Ⓒ Ⓓ	77. Ⓐ Ⓑ Ⓒ Ⓓ	87. Ⓐ Ⓑ Ⓒ Ⓓ
48. Ⓐ Ⓑ Ⓒ Ⓓ	58. Ⓐ Ⓑ Ⓒ Ⓓ	68. Ⓐ Ⓑ Ⓒ Ⓓ	78. Ⓐ Ⓑ Ⓒ Ⓓ	88. Ⓐ Ⓑ Ⓒ Ⓓ
49. Ⓐ Ⓑ Ⓒ Ⓓ	59. Ⓐ Ⓑ Ⓒ Ⓓ	69. Ⓐ Ⓑ Ⓒ Ⓓ	79. Ⓐ Ⓑ Ⓒ Ⓓ	89. Ⓐ Ⓑ Ⓒ Ⓓ
50. Ⓐ Ⓑ Ⓒ Ⓓ	60. Ⓐ Ⓑ Ⓒ Ⓓ	70. Ⓐ Ⓑ Ⓒ Ⓓ	80. Ⓐ Ⓑ Ⓒ Ⓓ	90. Ⓐ Ⓑ Ⓒ Ⓓ
51. Ⓐ Ⓑ Ⓒ Ⓓ	61. Ⓐ Ⓑ Ⓒ Ⓓ	71. Ⓐ Ⓑ Ⓒ Ⓓ	81. Ⓐ Ⓑ Ⓒ Ⓓ	91. Ⓐ Ⓑ Ⓒ Ⓓ
52. Ⓐ Ⓑ Ⓒ Ⓓ	62. Ⓐ Ⓑ Ⓒ Ⓓ	72. Ⓐ Ⓑ Ⓒ Ⓓ	82. Ⓐ Ⓑ Ⓒ Ⓓ	92. Ⓐ Ⓑ Ⓒ Ⓓ
53. Ⓐ Ⓑ Ⓒ Ⓓ	63. Ⓐ Ⓑ Ⓒ Ⓓ	73. Ⓐ Ⓑ Ⓒ Ⓓ	83. Ⓐ Ⓑ Ⓒ Ⓓ	93. Ⓐ Ⓑ Ⓒ Ⓓ
54. Ⓐ Ⓑ Ⓒ Ⓓ	64. Ⓐ Ⓑ Ⓒ Ⓓ	74. Ⓐ Ⓑ Ⓒ Ⓓ	84. Ⓐ Ⓑ Ⓒ Ⓓ	94. Ⓐ Ⓑ Ⓒ Ⓓ
55. Ⓐ Ⓑ Ⓒ Ⓓ	65. Ⓐ Ⓑ Ⓒ Ⓓ	75. Ⓐ Ⓑ Ⓒ Ⓓ	85. Ⓐ Ⓑ Ⓒ Ⓓ	95. Ⓐ Ⓑ Ⓒ Ⓓ

Tear Here

Biology: 50 questions, #96–145

96. Ⓐ Ⓑ Ⓒ Ⓓ　　106. Ⓐ Ⓑ Ⓒ Ⓓ　　116. Ⓐ Ⓑ Ⓒ Ⓓ　　126. Ⓐ Ⓑ Ⓒ Ⓓ　　136. Ⓐ Ⓑ Ⓒ Ⓓ

97. Ⓐ Ⓑ Ⓒ Ⓓ　　107. Ⓐ Ⓑ Ⓒ Ⓓ　　117. Ⓐ Ⓑ Ⓒ Ⓓ　　127. Ⓐ Ⓑ Ⓒ Ⓓ　　137. Ⓐ Ⓑ Ⓒ Ⓓ

98. Ⓐ Ⓑ Ⓒ Ⓓ　　108. Ⓐ Ⓑ Ⓒ Ⓓ　　118. Ⓐ Ⓑ Ⓒ Ⓓ　　128. Ⓐ Ⓑ Ⓒ Ⓓ　　138. Ⓐ Ⓑ Ⓒ Ⓓ

99. Ⓐ Ⓑ Ⓒ Ⓓ　　109. Ⓐ Ⓑ Ⓒ Ⓓ　　119. Ⓐ Ⓑ Ⓒ Ⓓ　　129. Ⓐ Ⓑ Ⓒ Ⓓ　　139. Ⓐ Ⓑ Ⓒ Ⓓ

100. Ⓐ Ⓑ Ⓒ Ⓓ　　110. Ⓐ Ⓑ Ⓒ Ⓓ　　120. Ⓐ Ⓑ Ⓒ Ⓓ　　130. Ⓐ Ⓑ Ⓒ Ⓓ　　140. Ⓐ Ⓑ Ⓒ Ⓓ

101. Ⓐ Ⓑ Ⓒ Ⓓ　　111. Ⓐ Ⓑ Ⓒ Ⓓ　　121. Ⓐ Ⓑ Ⓒ Ⓓ　　131. Ⓐ Ⓑ Ⓒ Ⓓ　　141. Ⓐ Ⓑ Ⓒ Ⓓ

102. Ⓐ Ⓑ Ⓒ Ⓓ　　112. Ⓐ Ⓑ Ⓒ Ⓓ　　122. Ⓐ Ⓑ Ⓒ Ⓓ　　132. Ⓐ Ⓑ Ⓒ Ⓓ　　142. Ⓐ Ⓑ Ⓒ Ⓓ

103. Ⓐ Ⓑ Ⓒ Ⓓ　　113. Ⓐ Ⓑ Ⓒ Ⓓ　　123. Ⓐ Ⓑ Ⓒ Ⓓ　　133. Ⓐ Ⓑ Ⓒ Ⓓ　　143. Ⓐ Ⓑ Ⓒ Ⓓ

104. Ⓐ Ⓑ Ⓒ Ⓓ　　114. Ⓐ Ⓑ Ⓒ Ⓓ　　124. Ⓐ Ⓑ Ⓒ Ⓓ　　134. Ⓐ Ⓑ Ⓒ Ⓓ　　144. Ⓐ Ⓑ Ⓒ Ⓓ

105. Ⓐ Ⓑ Ⓒ Ⓓ　　115. Ⓐ Ⓑ Ⓒ Ⓓ　　125. Ⓐ Ⓑ Ⓒ Ⓓ　　135. Ⓐ Ⓑ Ⓒ Ⓓ　　145. Ⓐ Ⓑ Ⓒ Ⓓ

Quantitative Ability: 65 questions, #146–210

146. Ⓐ Ⓑ Ⓒ Ⓓ   159. Ⓐ Ⓑ Ⓒ Ⓓ   172. Ⓐ Ⓑ Ⓒ Ⓓ   185. Ⓐ Ⓑ Ⓒ Ⓓ   198. Ⓐ Ⓑ Ⓒ Ⓓ

147. Ⓐ Ⓑ Ⓒ Ⓓ   160. Ⓐ Ⓑ Ⓒ Ⓓ   173. Ⓐ Ⓑ Ⓒ Ⓓ   186. Ⓐ Ⓑ Ⓒ Ⓓ   199. Ⓐ Ⓑ Ⓒ Ⓓ

148. Ⓐ Ⓑ Ⓒ Ⓓ   161. Ⓐ Ⓑ Ⓒ Ⓓ   174. Ⓐ Ⓑ Ⓒ Ⓓ   187. Ⓐ Ⓑ Ⓒ Ⓓ   200. Ⓐ Ⓑ Ⓒ Ⓓ

149. Ⓐ Ⓑ Ⓒ Ⓓ   162. Ⓐ Ⓑ Ⓒ Ⓓ   175. Ⓐ Ⓑ Ⓒ Ⓓ   188. Ⓐ Ⓑ Ⓒ Ⓓ   201. Ⓐ Ⓑ Ⓒ Ⓓ

150. Ⓐ Ⓑ Ⓒ Ⓓ   163. Ⓐ Ⓑ Ⓒ Ⓓ   176. Ⓐ Ⓑ Ⓒ Ⓓ   189. Ⓐ Ⓑ Ⓒ Ⓓ   202. Ⓐ Ⓑ Ⓒ Ⓓ

151. Ⓐ Ⓑ Ⓒ Ⓓ   164. Ⓐ Ⓑ Ⓒ Ⓓ   177. Ⓐ Ⓑ Ⓒ Ⓓ   190. Ⓐ Ⓑ Ⓒ Ⓓ   203. Ⓐ Ⓑ Ⓒ Ⓓ

152. Ⓐ Ⓑ Ⓒ Ⓓ   165. Ⓐ Ⓑ Ⓒ Ⓓ   178. Ⓐ Ⓑ Ⓒ Ⓓ   191. Ⓐ Ⓑ Ⓒ Ⓓ   204. Ⓐ Ⓑ Ⓒ Ⓓ

153. Ⓐ Ⓑ Ⓒ Ⓓ   166. Ⓐ Ⓑ Ⓒ Ⓓ   179. Ⓐ Ⓑ Ⓒ Ⓓ   192. Ⓐ Ⓑ Ⓒ Ⓓ   205. Ⓐ Ⓑ Ⓒ Ⓓ

154. Ⓐ Ⓑ Ⓒ Ⓓ   167. Ⓐ Ⓑ Ⓒ Ⓓ   180. Ⓐ Ⓑ Ⓒ Ⓓ   193. Ⓐ Ⓑ Ⓒ Ⓓ   206. Ⓐ Ⓑ Ⓒ Ⓓ

155. Ⓐ Ⓑ Ⓒ Ⓓ   168. Ⓐ Ⓑ Ⓒ Ⓓ   181. Ⓐ Ⓑ Ⓒ Ⓓ   194. Ⓐ Ⓑ Ⓒ Ⓓ   207. Ⓐ Ⓑ Ⓒ Ⓓ

156. Ⓐ Ⓑ Ⓒ Ⓓ   169. Ⓐ Ⓑ Ⓒ Ⓓ   182. Ⓐ Ⓑ Ⓒ Ⓓ   195. Ⓐ Ⓑ Ⓒ Ⓓ   208. Ⓐ Ⓑ Ⓒ Ⓓ

157. Ⓐ Ⓑ Ⓒ Ⓓ   170. Ⓐ Ⓑ Ⓒ Ⓓ   183. Ⓐ Ⓑ Ⓒ Ⓓ   196. Ⓐ Ⓑ Ⓒ Ⓓ   209. Ⓐ Ⓑ Ⓒ Ⓓ

158. Ⓐ Ⓑ Ⓒ Ⓓ   171. Ⓐ Ⓑ Ⓒ Ⓓ   184. Ⓐ Ⓑ Ⓒ Ⓓ   197. Ⓐ Ⓑ Ⓒ Ⓓ   210. Ⓐ Ⓑ Ⓒ Ⓓ

Tear Here

Chemistry: 60 questions, #211–270

211. Ⓐ Ⓑ Ⓒ Ⓓ   223. Ⓐ Ⓑ Ⓒ Ⓓ   235. Ⓐ Ⓑ Ⓒ Ⓓ   247. Ⓐ Ⓑ Ⓒ Ⓓ   259. Ⓐ Ⓑ Ⓒ Ⓓ

212. Ⓐ Ⓑ Ⓒ Ⓓ   224. Ⓐ Ⓑ Ⓒ Ⓓ   236. Ⓐ Ⓑ Ⓒ Ⓓ   248. Ⓐ Ⓑ Ⓒ Ⓓ   260. Ⓐ Ⓑ Ⓒ Ⓓ

213. Ⓐ Ⓑ Ⓒ Ⓓ   225. Ⓐ Ⓑ Ⓒ Ⓓ   237. Ⓐ Ⓑ Ⓒ Ⓓ   249. Ⓐ Ⓑ Ⓒ Ⓓ   261. Ⓐ Ⓑ Ⓒ Ⓓ

214. Ⓐ Ⓑ Ⓒ Ⓓ   226. Ⓐ Ⓑ Ⓒ Ⓓ   238. Ⓐ Ⓑ Ⓒ Ⓓ   250. Ⓐ Ⓑ Ⓒ Ⓓ   262. Ⓐ Ⓑ Ⓒ Ⓓ

215. Ⓐ Ⓑ Ⓒ Ⓓ   227. Ⓐ Ⓑ Ⓒ Ⓓ   239. Ⓐ Ⓑ Ⓒ Ⓓ   251. Ⓐ Ⓑ Ⓒ Ⓓ   263. Ⓐ Ⓑ Ⓒ Ⓓ

216. Ⓐ Ⓑ Ⓒ Ⓓ   228. Ⓐ Ⓑ Ⓒ Ⓓ   240. Ⓐ Ⓑ Ⓒ Ⓓ   252. Ⓐ Ⓑ Ⓒ Ⓓ   264. Ⓐ Ⓑ Ⓒ Ⓓ

217. Ⓐ Ⓑ Ⓒ Ⓓ   229. Ⓐ Ⓑ Ⓒ Ⓓ   241. Ⓐ Ⓑ Ⓒ Ⓓ   253. Ⓐ Ⓑ Ⓒ Ⓓ   265. Ⓐ Ⓑ Ⓒ Ⓓ

218. Ⓐ Ⓑ Ⓒ Ⓓ   230. Ⓐ Ⓑ Ⓒ Ⓓ   242. Ⓐ Ⓑ Ⓒ Ⓓ   254. Ⓐ Ⓑ Ⓒ Ⓓ   266. Ⓐ Ⓑ Ⓒ Ⓓ

219. Ⓐ Ⓑ Ⓒ Ⓓ   231. Ⓐ Ⓑ Ⓒ Ⓓ   243. Ⓐ Ⓑ Ⓒ Ⓓ   255. Ⓐ Ⓑ Ⓒ Ⓓ   267. Ⓐ Ⓑ Ⓒ Ⓓ

220. Ⓐ Ⓑ Ⓒ Ⓓ   232. Ⓐ Ⓑ Ⓒ Ⓓ   244. Ⓐ Ⓑ Ⓒ Ⓓ   256. Ⓐ Ⓑ Ⓒ Ⓓ   268. Ⓐ Ⓑ Ⓒ Ⓓ

221. Ⓐ Ⓑ Ⓒ Ⓓ   233. Ⓐ Ⓑ Ⓒ Ⓓ   245. Ⓐ Ⓑ Ⓒ Ⓓ   257. Ⓐ Ⓑ Ⓒ Ⓓ   269. Ⓐ Ⓑ Ⓒ Ⓓ

222. Ⓐ Ⓑ Ⓒ Ⓓ   234. Ⓐ Ⓑ Ⓒ Ⓓ   246. Ⓐ Ⓑ Ⓒ Ⓓ   258. Ⓐ Ⓑ Ⓒ Ⓓ   270. Ⓐ Ⓑ Ⓒ Ⓓ

READING COMPREHENSION

Number of Questions: 45
Time: 45 MINUTES

Directions: Read each of the following five passages and choose the best answer to the questions that follow each passage. There is only one correct answer for each question.

Questions 1–8 are based on the following passage.

Anatomy of Swallowing

Line   Dysphagia, assumes many forms; the anatomy and mechanics of swallowing demonstrate why. Fifty pairs of muscles maneuver through a series of voluntary and involuntary neuromuscular contractions as food is chewed and moves from the mouth to the stomach. This process has three distinct phases:

    1. Preparation and oral stage. As food is chewed, the mouth manipulates food and liquid. The tongue
(5)   propels food and liquid to the back of the mouth, starting the swallowing response.

    2. Oropharyngeal stage. During this stage, food and liquid quickly pass through the pharynx, the canal that connects the mouth to the esophagus. Various muscles steer food or drink to the esophagus's opening. The larynx, meanwhile, closes tightly and breathing momentarily stops, preventing food and liquid from entering the lungs.

(10) 3. Esophageal stage. The average esophagus is about 9 to 10 inches long and about 1.2 inches wide. Food and liquid pass through the upper esophageal sphincter, a one-way valve to the esophagus. Peristaltic waves propel food down the esophagus, taking as long as 20 seconds, depending on the food's texture and consistency. When the lower esophageal sphincter relaxes and the food or liquid enters the stomach, swallowing is complete. While people have some voluntary control over the first
(15)   stage, the oropharyngeal and esophageal stages occur involuntarily. A change in any part of these intricate swallowing processes can lead to dysphagia.

Dysphagia Subtypes

    The vast majority of disorders occur in the involuntary stage 2 (oropharyngeal dysphagia) and stage 3 (esoph-
(20) ageal dysphagia).

    Oropharyngeal dysphagia impairs either food transport to the back of the mouth or initiation of the swallowing reflex, thus creating a dysfunctional transfer of food and liquid through the pharynx, past the upper esophageal sphincter, and into the esophagus. People with this type of dysphagia frequently complain that food "sticks" in the throat; they may also choke, cough, or experience nasal regurgitation during swallowing. Oropharyngeal dysphagia
(25) is the most common subtype observed among the elderly, particularly among stroke victims.

    Three problems lead to esophageal dysphagia: impaired esophageal peristaltic motility, esophageal obstruction, and stomach acid reflux into the esophagus. Occasional acid reflux is uncomfortable, but consistent reflux can inflame and narrow the esophagus. Chest discomfort shortly after swallowing is esophageal dysphagia's hallmark.

Reprinted with permission from Consultant Pharmacist, *Vol. 18, No. 1, January 2003, Pages 14–15.*

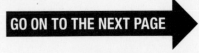
GO ON TO THE NEXT PAGE

1. Which of the following problems does NOT lead to esophageal dysphagia?

    (A) Impaired esophageal peristaltic motility

    (B) Renal obstruction

    (C) Esophageal obstruction

    (D) Stomach acid reflux into the esophagus

2. The average esophagus is approximately

    (A) 2-4 inches long.

    (B) 5-8 inches long.

    (C) 9-10 inches long.

    (D) 11-14 inches long.

3. _____ _____of muscles maneuver through a series of voluntary and involuntary neuromuscular contractions as food is chewed and moves from the mouth to the stomach.

    (A) Twenty pairs

    (B) Thirty pairs

    (C) Forty pairs

    (D) Fifty pairs

4. The_____is the canal that connects the mouth to the esophagus.

    (A) pharynx

    (B) canal of Schlemm

    (C) Inner canal

    (D) Outer canal

5. Dysphagia disorders occur most frequently during which stages of swallowing?

    (A) One and three

    (B) One and four

    (C) Two and three

    (D) One and two

6. _____dysphagia is the most common subtype observed among the elderly, particularly among stroke victims.

    (A) Esophageal

    (B) Oropharyngeal

    (C) Pharyngeal

    (D) Reflux

7. Food and liquid pass through the upper esophageal sphincter, a_____valve to the esophagus.

    (A) one-way

    (B) two-way

    (C) single

    (D) narrow

8. The_____ closes tightly and breathing momentarily stops, preventing food and liquid from entering the lungs.

    (A) esophagus

    (B) throat

    (C) oropharyngeal canal

    (D) larynx

Questions 9–18 are based on the following passage.

Use of Botulinum Toxin Type B for Migraine and Tension Headaches

Line   Headache is the most common patient complaint reported to health-care professionals. During the past twenty
years, there has been heated debate as to whether primary headaches (such as tension headache, migraine headache, cluster headache, and rebound headache secondary to analgesic abuse) are neurogenic or vascular in origin.
Current molecular and functional studies suggest a way of combining both neurologic and vascular causes of
(5)   headaches.

Botulinum toxin type B, a neurotoxin produced by Clostridium botulinum, acts by blocking acetylcholine release at the neuromuscular junction. Botulinum toxin type B, unlike botulinum toxin type A, is available as a sterile
solution for injection of a purified neurotoxin produced by fermentation of the bacterium. Because of differences
in vehicles, dilution schemes, and laboratory protocols for determining the median lethal dose in mice, units of
(10) biological activity of botulinum toxin type B cannot be directly converted into units of activity of other types of
botulinum toxin. However, botulinum toxin type B 5,000 units/ml. is generally considered to have a therapeutic
effect similar to that of botulinum toxin type A 100 units/ml. Therefore, botulinum toxin type B may offer benefits
to patients for whom we would otherwise use low-dose botulinum toxin type A.

Injectable botulinum toxin type B solution (Myobloc, South San Francisco, CA) was used at a neurology clinic as
(15) an adjunctive therapy for two patients with refractory headaches. One patient had migraine headache, and, the
other, muscle-tension headache. The frequency of headaches was noted each week after treatment. The severity of
headaches was recorded by the patient on a scale from 0–5, where 0 = no headache and 5 = severe headache,
before and after treatment. Botulinum toxin type B was given every three months. The use of prescription pain
relievers was also recorded. These two patients were chosen at random by the neurologist at our neurology clinic
(20) to receive botulinum toxin type B.

Reprinted with permission from American Journal of Health Systems Pharmacist, *Vol. 59, October 1, 2002, Page 1,860.*

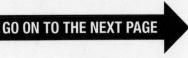

9. What is the trade name of botulinum toxin type B solution?

(A) Botutoc

(B) Toxbloc

(C) Myobloc

(D) Botubloc

10. The mechanism of action of botulinum toxin type B is to block

(A) acetylcholine release.

(B) acetylcholine release at the neuromuscular junction.

(C) norepinephrine release at the neuromuscular junction.

(D) choline release at the neuromuscular junction.

11. Which of the following is available in a sterile solution?

(A) Toxin type A

(B) Toxin type B

(C) Toxin type C

(D) Toxin type D

12. According to this passage, what is the most common patient complaint reported to health-care professionals?

(A) Dizziness

(B) Headache

(C) Blurred vision

(D) Dry mouth

13. Which of the following is NOT a reason why botulinum toxin type B cannot be converted into units?

(A) Dilution schemes

(B) Differences in vehicles

(C) Differences in preservatives

(D) Laboratory protocols

14. The scale used in the passage to measure severity of the headache was characterized by

(A) 0 = severe headache.

(B) 5 = severe headache.

(C) 4 = moderate headache.

(D) 3 = not sure.

15. According to the passage, primary headaches include all of the following EXCEPT

(A) tension headache.

(B) cluster headache.

(C) molecular headache.

(D) migraine headache.

16. How often was botulinum toxin type B administered in this study?

(A) Every two months

(B) Every three months

(C) Every four months

(D) Every five months

17. _____units/ml. of botulinum toxin type B are similar to _____ units/ml. of botulinum toxin type A.

(A) 2,500; 250

(B) 1,500; 100

(C) 4,000; 100

(D) 5,000; 100

18. According to this passage, Myobloc was used at a

(A) cardiovascular clinic.

(B) surgery.

(C) neurology.

(D) opthamology.

Questions 19–30 are based on the following passage.

Knocking Down Genes for Fun and Function

Line   Scientists once thought of eukaryotic RNA as solely active in transcription as messenger RNA (mRNA), and in translation as transfer RNA (tRNA). After Fire and colleagues first reported that double-stranded RNA (dsRNA) can interfere with gene expression, the conception of how gene transcription works was knocked on its head. Suddenly, these pieces of RNA, which appeared to be cellular detritus sliced out of mRNA, took on importance: They
(5)   could have a role in gene suppression.

Subsequent papers by many groups, including these two Hot Papers by Thomas Tuschl and colleagues, formerly of the Max Planck Institute for Biophysical Chemistry in Gottingen, Germany, clarify how the naturally occurring method of RNA inhibition works, and how engineered small inhibitory RNAs (siRNAs) can be introduced into a cell to knock down, or suppress, specific gene expression. Barely five years since the concept was first published,
(10)   researchers are looking to use siRNAs clinically.

The first paper, Tuschl explains, "is the formal proof that siRNA can do gene silencing." The second paper, he says, shows that siRNAs can direct gene silencing in mammalian cells without interference that kills the cells.

CRUCIAL INFORMATION: In a naturally occurring system, posttranscriptional gene silencing (PTGS) may be a means of protecting cells from transposons or viruses that can produce dsRNA. Within the cell, these dsRNAs are
(15)   enzymatically cut into smaller RNA pieces, which then bind to homologous mRNA, preventing translation of certain gene products. RNA fragments longer than about 30 nucleotides may destroy cellular mRNA, resulting in cytotoxicity and apoptosis.

But Tuschl's group, using a *Drosophila* lysate system, showed that RNAi—the suppression of gene expression by RNA fragments—occurs when the RNA fragments are 21- or 22-nucleotide duplexes of sense and antisense RNA.
(20)   These fragments are broken down from the dsRNA by the Dicer enzyme. Tuschl and colleagues identified efficacious segment lengths for PTGS using synthesized siRNA artificially introduced into cells.

Identifying the siRNA lengths that best suppressed gene expression in an in vitro *Drosophila* system was helpful in studies of invertebrate and plant systems, but methods for successfully using these extrinsic siRNAs in mammalian systems were elusive. Tuschl says that geneticists discovered the RNA silencing system, but "there was no
(25)   biochemical system that showed [how] a specific long RNA is degraded" to siRNA. Brenda Bass, a Howard Hughes Medical Institute investigator at University of Utah, Salt Lake City, notes that "conventional methods of initiating RNAi with long double-stranded RNA do not work in most mammalian cells." The key to inhibition of mammalian gene expression was found in the shorter siRNA segments.

Nearly two years ago, Tuschl's team reported on the successful use of extrinsic siRNAs in a mammalian cell
(30)   culture system. "Once we showed how it worked in flies… we could go into mammalian cells and see if we…[could] silence a gene," says Tuschl. They could. "This paper provided the crucial information that allowed researchers to use RNA interference in mammalian cells," explains Bass, who wrote a commentary on the Nature paper. "This paper showed that … an intermediate in the RNAi pathway (siRNA), could be successfully used to initiate RNAi in mammalian cells."

Reprinted with permission from The Scientist, *January 13, 2003, Pages 36-37.*

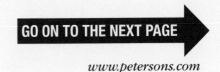

19. Tuschl said that this is the_____paper "that is formal proof that siRNA can do gene silencing."

    (A) fourth
    (B) third
    (C) second
    (D) first

20. What is a siRNA?

    (A) Small initial RNA
    (B) Small inhibitory RNA
    (C) Sense inhibitory RNA
    (D) Sense initial RNA

21. Who first reported that double-stranded RNA could interfere with gene expression?

    (A) Fire and colleagues
    (B) Frist and colleagues
    (C) Free and colleagues
    (D) Frost and colleagues

22. What lysate system did Tuschl's group utilize in this study?

    (A) Drosophagia
    (B) Drisophagia
    (C) Drosophela
    (D) Drosophila

23. Which of the following did Tuschl and colleagues identify in this study?

    (A) Widths of siRNA
    (B) Lengths of siRNA
    (C) Lengths of mRNA
    (D) Lengths of tRNA

24. What is PTGS?

    (A) Posttranscriptional gene silencing
    (B) Posttranscriptional gene splicing
    (C) Posttranscriptional gene sensing
    (D) Posttranscriptional gene solutions

25. Where was the key to inhibition of mammalian gene expression found according to this passage?

    (A) Shorter iRNA segments
    (B) Shorter sRNA segments
    (C) Shorter siRNA segments
    (D) Shorter mRNA segments

26. What can cause direct gene silencing in mammalian cells without interference that kills the cells?

    (A) mRNA
    (B) siRNA
    (C) iRNA
    (D) siDNA

27. How many fragments of nucleoxide duplexes of sense and antisense RNA are necessary for the suppression of gene expression by RNA?

    (A) 20 or 22
    (B) 19 or 20
    (C) 21 or 23
    (D) 21 or 22

28. What type of cells was used in this study?

    (A) Fly and mammalian cells
    (B) Fly cells
    (C) Mammalian cells
    (D) Cell cultures

29. What type of cells did Tuschl's group first work with before progressing to mammalian cells?

(A) Rats

(B) Flies

(C) Mice

(D) Guinea pigs

30. What type of pathway did the Nature manuscript show could be successful in initiating RNAi in mammalian cells?

(A) pRNA

(B) tRNA

(C) mRNA

(D) siRNA

GO ON TO THE NEXT PAGE

Questions 31–37 are based on the following passage.

Accelerating X-ray Crystallography

Line For years, the process of X-ray crystallography has moved at a tortoise's pace. "When I started in the field, it would typically take 20 person-years to produce a complete atomic model of one single protein. It was like a traffic jam in New York City. Every single part of the process was slow," says Stephen Burley, chief scientific officer and senior vice president of research at San Diego-based Structural GenomiX. The biggest holdup: obtaining a suitable
(5) crystal.

Researchers can spend weeks or even months searching for optimal crystallization conditions. "You need a crystal and without a crystal you have nothing to do," explains Tom Hurley, professor of biochemistry and molecular biology at Indiana University. Other bottlenecks include data collection and data analysis.

Now the biotech industry and some academics are trying to kick the process up to hare speed. New high-
(10) throughput (HT) methods being developed will dramatically improve the pace at which researchers collect and analyze data on larger and more poorly diffracting proteins, macromolecular complexes, and nucleic acids. This improvement will transform the labor-intensive and time-consuming process of molecular structure determination by X-ray crystallography into a powerful and viable method for advancing functional genomics, and ultimately, for translating raw genomic information into new pharmaceuticals.

(15) "The whole notion is to do more, faster, using automation as much as possible," explains Mark Rould, director of the University of Vermont's Center for X-ray Crystallography and assistant professor of molecular physiology and biophysics at the schools's college of medicine. "Crystallography has gone from solving a structure once every decade to solving 75 percent of the projects in the lab within a week of collecting the data," explains Hurley.

SCHOLARLY DEBATE: Not everyone agrees about the feasibility and benefits of HT X-ray crystallography; some
(20) consider the goal of Structural GenomiX—5,000 proteins in five years—overly ambitious. Crystallographer Gongyi Zhang, National Jewish Medical and Research Center and University of Colorado Health Sciences Center, Denver, says that crystallization was, is, and will continue to be a rate-limiting step. Eventually, he says, biotech companies will fail to keep the pace they have been bragging about. Hurley, who believes HT techniques "will lead to a huge explosion of understanding in biochemistry," says that considerable development is still needed before leaping
(25) from structural determination to drug design.

Reprinted from The Scientist, *January 13, 2003, Page 39.*

31. How many person-years did it take to produce a complete atomic model of a single protein?

    (A) Ten
    (B) Fifteen
    (C) Twenty
    (D) Twenty-five

32. According to this passage, what are two bottlenecks researchers must face when searching for optimal crystallization conditions?

    (A) Funds for research
    (B) Data collection
    (C) Data analysis
    (D) B and C

33. What does Gongyi Zhang say will continue to be a rate-limiting step?

    (A) Crystallization
    (B) Polymorphism
    (C) Cost of finding the best crystallization process
    (D) HT techniques

34. What does HT methods refer to?

    (A) High-temperature methods
    (B) High-throughput methods
    (C) Hard-throughput methods
    (D) High-theoretical methods

35. Crystallography has progressed from solving a structure once every decade to solving _____ of the projects.

    (A) 25 percent
    (B) 50 percent
    (C) 70 percent
    (D) 75 percent

36. According to Stephen Burley, chief scientific officer of Structural GenomiX, the biggest holdup is obtaining a suitable

    (A) crystal.
    (B) molecule.
    (C) atom.
    (D) ion.

37. The improvements in the process of molecular structure determination by X-ray crystallography will ultimately result in translation of

    (A) raw genomic information into new pharmaceuticals.
    (B) crystallization information into new pharmaceuticals.
    (C) raw genetic information into new pharmaceuticals.
    (D) raw information into new pharmaceuticals.

GO ON TO THE NEXT PAGE

Questions 38–45 are based on the following passage.

Crystal Structure of *Escherichia coli* MscS, a Voltage-Modulated and Mechanosensitive Channel

Line   The mechanosensitive channel of small conductance, MscS, was identified by Kung and coworkers as a stretch-activated channel present in the inner membrane of *E. coli*. The MscS channel is characterized by a conductance of ~1 nS, with a slight preference for anions; this is substantially larger than the conductances of typical eukaryotic ion channels (1 to 30 pS), but smaller than the ~3 nS, nonselective conductance observed for the prokaryotic MscL

(5)   (large conductance) mechanosensitive channel. Both MscS and MscL are intrinsically mechanosensitive, opening in response to stretching of the cell membrane without the requisite participation of cytoskeletal or other components. The pressure threshold for MscS opening is ~50 percent that of MscL, which in turn opens at pressures near the rupture point of the bilayer. The properties of these channels likely reflect their involvement in the cellular response to rapid decreases in external osmolarity, and the two channels share the ability to partially compensate

(10)   for the deletion of the other. The gene encoding the MscS channel, yggB, was identified by Booth and co-workers; the *E. coli* protein, with 286 amino acids is predicted from hydropathy analyses to have three transmembrane helices and exhibits no detectable sequence similarities to the smaller (136 residues) MscL. In common with MscL and other prokaryotic channels, such as KcsA, MscS exists as a homo-oligomer. However, MscS has a far greater distribution than MscL throughout eubacteria, and has also been identified in Archaea and at least some eukaryotes.

(15)   The conductances of gated channels such as MscS are regulated by conformational switching of the protein structure between open and closed states. This switching responds to changes in environmental conditions, including applied tension (mechanosensitive channels), variation in membrane potential (voltage-gated channels), and binding of ligands (ligand-gated channels). In recent years, progress has been made in defining the structural basis of channel gating. After the structure of the closed state of MscL was determined, detailed models were described

(20)   for the structure of the open state and the coupling between membrane tension and structure. Structural aspects of the mechanism of ligand gating have been established for opening a prokaryotic potassium channel by proton binding to the channel and by calcium binding to an extramembrane domain. Although considerable insights into the mechanism of voltage-dependent gating have been achieved, to date, no structures of a voltage-gated system have been described.

Reprinted with permission from Science, *Vol. 298, November 22, 2002, Page 1,582, American Association for the Advancement of Science.*

38. The conductances of gated channels such as_____are regulated by conformational switching of the protein structure between open and closed states.

    (A) KcsA

    (B) MscS

    (C) MscL

    (D) mRNA

39. A mechanosenstive channel of small conductance is known as

    (A) MscL.

    (B) mRNA.

    (C) KcsA.

    (D) MscS.

40. MscS channel is characterized by a conductance of

    (A) ~ 1 nS.

    (B) ~ 2 nS.

    (C) ~ 3 nS.

    (D) ~ 4 nS.

41. Which of the following best describes the status of structures of a voltage-gated system?

    (A) Three structures have been described.

    (B) Two new structures have been described.

    (C) One new structure has been described.

    (D) No structures have been described.

42. Both MscS and MscL are_____ mechanosensitive.

    (A) extrinsically

    (B) intrinsically

    (C) extrinsically and intrinsically

    (D) less mechanosensitive than KscL

43. Which of the following best describes the structural aspects of the mechanism of ligand gating established for opening a prokaryotic potassium channel by proton binding to the channel and by calcium binding to an extramembrane domain?

    (A) Protein binding to the channel

    (B) Peptide binding to the channel

    (C) Proton binding to the channel

    (D) Protase binding to the channel

44. According to this passage, how many amino acids does the *E. coli* have?

    (A) 236 amino acids

    (B) 286 amino acids

    (C) 256 amino acids

    (D) 268 amino acids

45. What is the pressure threshold for MscS compared to that of MscL?

    (A) ~ 20 percent of that of MscL

    (B) ~ 30 percent of that of MscL

    (C) ~ 40 percent of that of MscL

    (D) ~ 50 percent of that of MscL

STOP If you finish before time is called, you may check your work on this section only. Do not turn to any other section in the test.

VERBAL ABILITY

Number of Questions: 50
Time: 30 MINUTES

Directions: For questions 46–70, choose the lettered word that means the *opposite* or *most nearly the opposite* as the word in capital letters. There is only one correct answer for each question.

46. EXISTENCE
- (A) life
- (B) reality
- (C) actuality
- (D) nonexistence

47. KNOWABLE
- (A) fathomable
- (B) unknowable
- (C) understandable
- (D) graspable

48. INTERFUSION
- (A) mixture
- (B) splitting
- (C) combination
- (D) blending

49. INTIMATE
- (A) stranger
- (B) mate
- (C) confidant
- (D) associate

50. METAMORPHOSE
- (A) commute
- (B) transmogrify
- (C) static
- (D) transform

51. OUTCRY
- (A) upheaval
- (B) commotion
- (C) clamor
- (D) acquiescence

52. RUBBISH
- (A) nonsense
- (B) factual
- (C) kelter
- (D) bilge

53. SHANTY
- (A) estate
- (B) abode
- (C) shaker
- (D) shack

54. ABDICATION
- (A) resignation
- (B) enlistment
- (C) abandonment
- (D) departed

55. ASCRIBE
- (A) abstain
- (B) attribute
- (C) impute
- (D) assign

56. CREDIBLE
- **(A)** logical
- **(B)** authentic
- **(C)** believable
- **(D)** distrust

57. PERENNIALLY
- **(A)** annually
- **(B)** constantly
- **(C)** perpetually
- **(D)** continuously

58. EMINENCE
- **(A)** level
- **(B)** protuberance
- **(C)** steep
- **(D)** loftiness

59. TANGLE
- **(A)** untangle
- **(B)** involve
- **(C)** hamper
- **(D)** complicate

60. CAVILING
- **(A)** appreciative
- **(B)** arguing
- **(C)** quibbling
- **(D)** finding fault

61. DECLINATION
- **(A)** ascension
- **(B)** deterioration
- **(C)** obliquity
- **(D)** deviation

62. EMANATE
- **(A)** radiate
- **(B)** emerge
- **(C)** result
- **(D)** rescind

63. DEFENSIBLE
- **(A)** indefensible
- **(B)** justifiable
- **(C)** just
- **(D)** defendable

64. EMPIRICAL
- **(A)** experimental
- **(B)** probative
- **(C)** tentative
- **(D)** absolute

65. EYEWASH
- **(A)** collyrium
- **(B)** humbuggery
- **(C)** truth
- **(D)** bunkum

66. PURPOSELESS
- **(A)** uncertain
- **(B)** random
- **(C)** unordered
- **(D)** directed

67. GENIALITY
- **(A)** cordiality
- **(B)** rudeness
- **(C)** hospitality
- **(D)** cheerfulness

GO ON TO THE NEXT PAGE

68. HARNESS

(A) armor

(B) parachute

(C) unprotected

(D) wardrobe

69. HYPOTHESIS

(A) fact

(B) premise

(C) theory

(D) supposition

70. IMPONDERABLE

(A) immaterial

(B) infinitesimal

(C) ponderable

(D) unweighable

Directions: For questions 71–95, select the word that best completes the analogy. There is only one correct answer.

71. LIBELOUS : CALUMNIOUS :: APPLAUDING :

(A) adulating

(B) invidious

(C) traducing

(D) detracting

72. MATRIARCH : DOWAGER :: DIVORCE :

(A) dame

(B) elope

(C) dowry

(D) sunder

73. PHYSICIAN : SAWBONES :: PHARMACIST :

(A) surgeon

(B) doc

(C) apothecary

(D) physic

74. PILASTER : COLUMN :: DOCK :

(A) pier

(B) pile

(C) boat

(D) piffle

75. ENCUMBERANCE : IMPEDANCE :: RESULT :

(A) assist

(B) assistance

(C) catalyst

(D) sequence

76. FERINE : BESTIAL :: FERTILE :

(A) fecund

(B) infertile

(C) sterile

(D) animal

77. CARBUNCLE : FURUNCLE :: AUBERGE :

(A) carburetor

(B) caravansary

(C) dimple

(D) doldrum

78. DEARTH : ABSENCE :: DEAN :

(A) leader

(B) follower

(C) professor

(D) actor

79. ENGROSS : DISPERSE :: ENGAGING :

(A) gross

(B) bewilder

(C) loathsome

(D) inscribe

80. FANCIER : AMATEUR :: WALLFLOWER :
- **(A)** dancer
- **(B)** imaginary
- **(C)** enthusiast
- **(D)** caprice

81. OYSTER : FORTE :: JOHN DORY :
- **(A)** shrimp
- **(B)** lobster
- **(C)** crab
- **(D)** fish

82. SLEIGHT : ADROITNESS :: MENIAL :
- **(A)** dray horse
- **(B)** pony
- **(C)** mule
- **(D)** bay

83. TREATISE : MONOGRAPH :: AGREEMENT :
- **(A)** contract
- **(B)** vows
- **(C)** dissent
- **(D)** telegraph

84. VORACIOUS : EDACIOUS :: VORTEX :
- **(A)** bodacious
- **(B)** maelstrom
- **(C)** vulturous
- **(D)** votary

85. WAGGERY : EARNEST :: WAGGLE :
- **(A)** switch
- **(B)** vulpine
- **(C)** impishness
- **(D)** ludicrous

86. LEXICON : WORDSTOCK :: LIAR :
- **(A)** honest
- **(B)** wordy
- **(C)** wordsmith
- **(D)** perjurer

87. TACIT : EXPLICIT :: TACKY :
- **(A)** expressed
- **(B)** implicit
- **(C)** categorical
- **(D)** modish

88. XANTHIPPE : SHREW :: WRECKAGE :
- **(A)** sabotage
- **(B)** shred
- **(C)** screen
- **(D)** sardonic

89. ZANY : HARLEQUIN :: THESPIAN :
- **(A)** buffoon
- **(B)** mummer
- **(C)** drummer
- **(D)** theatric

90. UTTERANCE : SILENCE :: ANNIHILATE :
- **(A)** abolish
- **(B)** extirpate
- **(C)** invent
- **(D)** salient

91. SLOTH : SEDULITY :: HARE :
- **(A)** assiduity
- **(B)** assiduousness
- **(C)** diligence
- **(D)** slowpoke

GO ON TO THE NEXT PAGE

92. RUMINATE : MEDIATE :: RECREANT :

(A) perfidious

(B) recreate

(C) revolve

(D) revolt

93. POLITIC : EXPEDIENT :: POLITY :

(A) course

(B) tact

(C) polar

(D) civil

94. IRKSOME : ENGROSSING :: IRASCIBLE :

(A) exciting

(B) tolerant

(C) hateful

(D) tiresome

95. HONED : KEEN :: HORRID :

(A) lurid

(B) lean

(C) mean

(D) hewn

STOP   If you finish before time is called, you may check your work on this section only. Do not turn to any other section in the test.

BIOLOGY

Number of Questions: 50
Time: 30 MINUTES

Directions: For questions 96–145, select the correct answer and mark it on your answer sheet. There is only one correct answer for each question.

96. Which of the following is not an example of an exocrine gland?

    (A) Merocrine

    (B) Halocrine

    (C) Endocrine

    (D) Apocrine

97. Which of the following is true regarding an animal cell membrane?

    (A) The interior is hydrophilic and the exterior is hydrophobic.

    (B) The interior is hydrophilic and the exterior is hydrophilic.

    (C) The interior is hydrophobic and the exterior is hydrophilic.

    (D) The interior is hydrophobic and the exterior is hydrophobic.

98. Which of the following is incorrect regarding membrane transport?

    (A) Simple diffusion involves movement of molecules from an area of high concentration to an area of lower concentration.

    (B) Facilitated diffusion is the ATP-dependent movement of molecules or ions against a concentration gradient.

    (C) Filtration is when water and solutes are forced (high to low concentration) through a membrane by hydrostatic pressure.

    (D) Osmosis is the diffusion of water molecules through a selectively permeable membrane.

99. Which of the following is incorrect regarding cutaneous sensation?

    (A) Meissner's corpuscles are responsible for light touch detection.

    (B) Pacinian corpuscles are located in dermal papillae.

    (C) Pacinian corpuscles are responsible for pressure detection.

    (D) Meissner's corpuscles are found in areas such as fingertips, palms, soles, and eyelids.

100. Which of the following is a function of the hormone calcitonin?

    (A) It causes a deposition of bone matrix by inhibiting bone resorption and increasing osteoblast activity.

    (B) It increases blood Ca^{++} via stimulation of bone resorption.

    (C) It is secreted by the parathyroid gland.

    (D) It promotes Ca^{++} reabsorption in the kidney tubules.

101. Which of the following allows for bone growth until adulthood?

    (A) Bone shaft

    (B) Periosteum

    (C) Bone marrow

    (D) Epiphyseal growth plate

GO ON TO THE NEXT PAGE

102. Which of the following is least involved with muscle contraction?

(A) ATP

(B) Calcium

(C) Actin

(D) Potassium

103. Which neurotransmitter is involved in muscle contraction?

(A) Acetylcholine

(B) Serotonin

(C) Dopamine

(D) GABA

104. Which of the following is true regarding cellular energetics?

(A) Aerobic glycolysis results in alcohol and lactic acid fermentation.

(B) Lactic acid buildup results in muscle soreness and fatigue.

(C) Cellular respiration results in 46 ATP molecules being produced from a single glucose molecule.

(D) Glycolysis is the anaerobic conversion of 6-carbon sugar (e.g., glucose) to two pyruvate molecules, resulting in the formation of ATP.

105. Regarding the structure and function of neurons, all of the following are true EXCEPT

(A) dendrites are neuron extensions that carry impulses to the cell body.

(B) axons are neuron extensions that carry impulses away from the cell body.

(C) Schwann cells in the central nervous system produce myelin.

(D) there is only one axon per neuron.

106. The distribution of ions across the cell membrane determines the resting membrane potential (RMP) of a neuron. Which of the following is incorrect regarding the RMP?

(A) K^+ is high inside the cell.

(B) Na^+ is high inside the cell.

(C) Cl^- is high outside the cell.

(D) The Na^+K^+–ATPase pump is responsible for maintaining the RMP.

107. Movement of impulses from one neuron to another is known as synaptic transmission. Which of the following best describes the synapse?

(A) The actual electrical impulse

(B) The junction between two neurons

(C) The terminal process of the neuron

(D) The hormone response for impulse transmission

108. Which of the following best describes the process by which continual stimulation of the postsynaptic membrane is prevented?

(A) Neurotransmitters are either destroyed by specific enzymes in the synaptic cleft or undergo reuptake into the presynaptic cleft.

(B) Neurotransmitters diffuse from the synaptic cleft.

(C) Neurotransmitters undergo non-enzymatic breakdown.

(D) Neurotransmitters are either destroyed by specific enzymes in the synaptic cleft or undergo reuptake into the postsynaptic cleft.

109. Which of the following is incorrect regarding sensory receptors?

    (A) Mechanoreceptors respond to changes in pressure.

    (B) Thermoreceptors are the only somatic sensory receptors that do not undergo sensory adaptation.

    (C) Photoreceptors respond to light.

    (D) Nociceptor stimulation gives rise to pain sensation.

110. Analgesics are commonly used to reduce pain and inflammation. Which of the following is NOT considered an analgesic?

    (A) Ibuprofen

    (B) Tylenol

    (C) Aspirin

    (D) Lipitor

111. Sensory information received by the five special senses (hearing, vision, equilibrium, taste, and smell) is relayed to the brain by specific cranial nerves (CNs). Which of the following sense : cranial nerve associations is incorrect?

    (A) Smell : CN I

    (B) Hearing : CN VIII

    (C) Sight : CN II

    (D) Taste : CN X

112. Hormones are blood-borne messengers of the endocrine system. Which of the following is NOT an endocrine gland?

    (A) Pituitary

    (B) Thymus

    (C) Sebaceous

    (D) Testes

113. The hypothalamus triggers hormone release from the anterior pituitary. Which of the following is secreted by the hypothalamus?

    (A) Adrenocorticotropin hormone

    (B) Anti-diuretic hormone

    (C) Oxytocin

    (D) Aldosterone

114. The pancreas functions as an exocrine and an endocrine gland. Which of the following best describes the endocrine gland function of the pancreas?

    (A) The endocrine glands of the pancreas are known as Peyer's Patches.

    (B) The endocrine glands of the pancreas are known as Islets of Langerhans.

    (C) Insulin produced by b-cells increases blood glucose levels.

    (D) Glucagon produced by a-cells decreases blood glucose levels.

115. Arteries carry blood from the heart, and veins carry blood to the heart. In general, which of the following is true regarding oxygen and carbon dioxide levels carried by blood vessels?

    (A) Arteries carry blood that is *high* in carbon dioxide and *low* in oxygen.

    (B) Veins carry blood that is *high* in oxygen and *low* in oxygen.

    (C) Arteries carry blood that is *high* in oxygen and *low* in carbon dioxide.

    (D) Veins carry blood that is *high* in oxygen and carbon monoxide.

116. Which of the following separates the right atrium and ventricle?

    (A) Aortic semilunar valve

    (B) Tricuspid valve

    (C) Pulmonary semilunar valve

    (D) Bicuspid valve

GO ON TO THE NEXT PAGE

117. Which of the following is known as the "pacemaker" of the heart?

    (A) Atrioventricular node

    (B) Purkinje fibers

    (C) Sinoatrial node

    (D) Atrioventricular bundle

118. Which of the following is NOT one of the three waves comprising a single heartbeat?

    (A) T wave

    (B) QRS complex

    (C) Z wave

    (D) P wave

119. Which of the following is incorrect regarding mean arterial blood pressure (MABP)?

    (A) MABP is maximum during systole.

    (B) MABP is minimum during diastole.

    (C) Normal MABP is 120 mm. Hg./80 mm. Hg.

    (D) Cardiac output is the product of heart rate and MABP.

120. Which of the following is NOT a hormone responsible for increasing blood pressure?

    (A) Epinephrine

    (B) Antidiruetic hormone

    (C) Aldosterone

    (D) Histamine

121. Which is neither a primary nor a secondary organ of the lymphatic system?

    (A) Thymus

    (B) Lymph nodes

    (C) T-cells

    (D) Spleen

122. Which of the following is NOT a function of the lymphatic system?

    (A) Prevent edema by returning excess interstitial fluid to the cardiovascular system

    (B) Return proteins that leak out of the blood vessel capillaries

    (C) Transport water-soluble vitamins from the gastrointestinal system to the blood stream

    (D) Transport foreign particles to the lymph nodes

123. Which of the following is the site of T-cell maturation?

    (A) Lymph node

    (B) Thymus

    (C) Red bone marrow

    (D) Spleen

124. Which of the following is NOT a component of the body's nonspecific immune response?

    (A) Inflammation

    (B) Fever

    (C) Phagocytosis

    (D) Antibodies

125. Which of the following cell types are considered antigen-presenting cells that trigger the specific immune response?

    (A) Macrophage

    (B) T-cell

    (C) B-cell

    (D) Neutrophil

126. B-cells secrete antibodies, known as immunoglobulins, which provide antibody-mediated immunity. Which of the following immunoglobulin is involved in the allergic reaction?

    (A) IgA
    (B) IgE
    (C) IgM
    (D) IgG

127. Which of the following is a function of salivary amylase?

    (A) Converts polysaccharides to disaccharides
    (B) Contracts gastroesophageal sphincter
    (C) Breaks down fats and triglycerides
    (D) Causes release of pancreatic juice into the duodenum

128. Which of the following is NOT a function of the liver?

    (A) Inactivates of toxins
    (B) Filters old blood cells
    (C) Produces and secretes bile
    (D) Stores and concentrates bile between meals

129. Which of the following is the site where a majority of nutrients are absorbed?

    (A) Stomach
    (B) Large intestine
    (C) Colon
    (D) Small intestine

130. Which of the following best describes tidal volume?

    (A) Maximum volume of air that a person can expire after maximal inspiration
    (B) Volume of air that can be forcibly expired after the resting tidal volume has been expired
    (C) Volume of air entering the lungs during a single inspiration
    (D) Volume of air that can be inspired over and above the resting tidal volume

131. Alveoli are microscopic air sacs found in the lung. Which of the following is incorrect regarding the alveoli?

    (A) Alveoli are comprised of Type I and II alveolar cells.
    (B) Type I alveolar cells secrete surfactant.
    (C) Surfactant acts to decrease surface tension, facilitating gas exchange.
    (D) Alveolar macrophages remove foreign particles from the air spaces.

132. In a mixture of gases, the pressure exerted by each gas is independent of the pressure exerted by others. This is known as

    (A) Boyle's Law.
    (B) Dalton's Law.
    (C) Beer's Law.
    (D) Logan's Law.

133. Oxygen is transported in the blood bound to which of the following proteins?

    (A) Hemoglobin
    (B) Albumin
    (C) Alpha-1 acid glycoprotein
    (D) Transcortin

GO ON TO THE NEXT PAGE

134. CO_2 produced by cellular respiration is enzymatically converted to carbonic acid, which rapidly dissociates to bicarbonate ion. The reaction is reversed in the lungs and CO_2 is expelled. Which of the following enzymes is crucial to this process?

(A) Monoamine oxidase

(B) Dopamine decarboxylase

(C) Carbonic anhydrase

(D) 11-beta hydroxysteroid dehydrogenase

135. Which of the following is responsible for regulation of red blood cell formation (erythropoiesis)?

(A) Aldosterone

(B) Erythropoietin

(C) Renin

(D) Angiotensin

136. Which of the following is NOT involved in urine formation?

(A) Filtration

(B) Secretion

(C) Reabsorption

(D) Micturition

137. Which of the following is considered the functional unit of the kidney?

(A) Cortex

(B) Nephron

(C) Medulla

(D) Loop of Henle

138. Which of the following is incorrect regarding the kidney's role in maintaining total body water balance?

(A) Sodium reabsorption is an active process.

(B) Hormonal control of sodium reabsorption occurs mainly in the loop of Henle.

(C) Potassium ions serve as the counter-ion for sodium reabsorption in tubular epithelial cells.

(D) The majority of sodium and water reabsorption occurs in the proximal tubule.

139. Which of the following is incorrect regarding meiosis?

(A) Meiosis is a type of cell division that results in the formation of gametes, with half the number of chromosomes as the parent cell.

(B) Human sex cells are diploid.

(C) Fertilization results in a diploid zygote.

(D) The genetic information found in chromosomes is known as DNA.

140. Which of the following is NOT a hormone involved in the development of sex characteristics?

(A) Estrogen

(B) Testosterone

(C) Follicular stimulating hormone

(D) Angiotensin

141. A mutation is an error found in the genetic code. Which of the following is the most common type of genetic variation?

(A) DNA insertion

(B) DNA deletion

(C) Single nucleotide polymorphism (SNP)

(D) Tandem repeat

142. Alleles are alternate forms of the same gene. For autosomal genes, we inherit one allele from our mother and one from our father. Regarding inheritance, which of the following is incorrect?

(A) Phenotype is the manifested or expressed trait.

(B) Genotype determines phenotype.

(C) Homozygous means that we have inherited identical alleles.

(D) Homozygotes and heterozygotes always display a different phenotype.

143. Thousands of chemical reactions occur throughout the body. Which of the following is incorrect regarding chemical reaction rates?

(A) Higher reactant concentrations result in a more rapid reaction rate.

(B) Higher required activation energy results in a more rapid reaction rate.

(C) Lower temperature results in a lower reaction rate.

(D) The presence of a catalyst results in a faster reaction rate.

144. Enzymes can be thought of as protein catalysts. Which of the following is incorrect regarding enzymes?

(A) An enzyme undergoes no net chemical change as a result of the reaction it catalyzes.

(B) An enzyme increases the rate of a reaction; however, it will not cause a reaction to occur that would not have occurred in its absence.

(C) An enzyme affects the rate at which equilibrium is achieved and can thereby change the final equilibrium.

(D) An enzyme lowers the activation energy.

145. The paradigm of molecular biology is the flow of genetic information from DNA to RNA and then to protein. Which of the following is incorrect regarding this paradigm?

(A) DNA is comprised of adenine, cytosine, thymine, and guanine.

(B) The ribosome is the site of protein synthesis.

(C) Messenger RNA carries the appropriate amino acid to the ribosome during protein synthesis.

(D) Transfer of information from the gene to messenger RNA is known as transcription.

STOP If you finish before time is called, you may check your work on this section only. Do not turn to any other section in the test.

QUANTITATIVE ABILITY

Number of Questions: 45
Time: 45 MINUTES

Directions: Select the best answer to the following questions. There is only one correct answer for each question.

146. $\dfrac{3}{5} \times \dfrac{6}{8} =$

(A) $\dfrac{9}{13}$

(B) $\dfrac{3}{8}$

(C) $\dfrac{9}{20}$

(D) $\dfrac{9}{40}$

147. $\dfrac{2}{3} \div \dfrac{4}{9} =$

(A) $\dfrac{3}{2}$

(B) $\dfrac{8}{27}$

(C) $\dfrac{6}{12}$

(D) $\dfrac{12}{18}$

148. $\dfrac{1}{3} + \dfrac{2}{8} =$

(A) $\dfrac{3}{8}$

(B) $\dfrac{7}{12}$

(C) $\dfrac{3}{11}$

(D) $\dfrac{16}{24}$

149. $\dfrac{12}{15} - \dfrac{4}{10} =$

(A) $\dfrac{8}{15}$

(B) $\dfrac{5}{10}$

(C) $\dfrac{2}{5}$

(D) $\dfrac{1}{2}$

150. $\left[\dfrac{4}{8} \times \dfrac{6}{12} \right] + \dfrac{1}{4} =$

(A) $\dfrac{1}{2}$

(B) $\dfrac{11}{24}$

(C) $\dfrac{25}{100}$

(D) $\dfrac{5}{20}$

151. $3.2 + 5.6 - 0.3 =$

(A) 9.1

(B) 12.1

(C) 5.8

(D) 8.5

152. $300 \times 0.5 + 500 \times 0.3 =$

(A) 800

(B) 300

(C) 250

(D) 400

153. $0.25 (5 + 3) + 4 =$

(A) 6

(B) 3

(C) 12

(D) 12.25

154. $\dfrac{(4+8)}{0.4} - 1 =$

(A) 30

(B) 3

(C) 11

(D) 29

155. $\dfrac{(15-3)}{(2+4)} \times 2.5 =$

(A) 4.25

(B) 5

(C) 6.25

(D) 2

156. Seventy-five percent =

(A) 0.075

(B) $\dfrac{3}{4}$

(C) 75

(D) 7.5

157. $\dfrac{3}{5} =$

(A) 75 percent

(B) 25 percent

(C) 60 percent

(D) 55 percent

158. Fifteen percent of 40 cookies =

(A) 6 cookies

(B) 15 cookies

(C) 30 cookies

(D) 20 cookies

159. $5^3 + 5 =$

(A) 20

(B) 125

(C) 650

(D) 130

160. $2^3 \times 2^2 =$

(A) 32

(B) 10

(C) 16

(D) 48

161. $Y^n \times Y^m =$

(A) $(n + m) \times Y$

(B) $Y^{(n + m)}$

(C) $Y^{(n \times m)}$

(D) $(n \times m) \times Y$

162. $X^2 \times Y^{-2} =$

(A) $(XY)^4$

(B) $(XY)^{-4}$

(C) $\dfrac{X^2}{Y^{\frac{1}{2}}}$

(D) $\dfrac{X^2}{Y^2}$

163. $\sqrt[3]{8} =$

(A) 24

(B) 512

(C) 3

(D) 2

164. $\sqrt{2} \times \sqrt{6} \times \sqrt{3} =$

(A) 24

(B) 12

(C) 6

(D) 3

GO ON TO THE NEXT PAGE ➤

165. $\log_5(25) =$

   (A) 5
   (B) 2
   (C) 1
   (D) 2.5

166. What is the common factor of 55 and 154?

   (A) 5
   (B) 7
   (C) 10
   (D) 11

167. Which of the following is a prime number?

   (A) 9
   (B) 0.5
   (C) 2^3
   (D) 11

168. Which of the following is NOT true?

   (A) $23 > 33 - 12$
   (B) $7 < 49^{\frac{1}{2}}$
   (C) $25 \geq 5^2$
   (D) $16 \leq 2 \times 9$

169. $13 - |-2| + |-6| =$

   (A) 17
   (B) 5
   (C) 1
   (D) 21

170. The expression: $5 \times [25 \times 8 \times (3+4)] = (5 \times 25) \times 8 \times (3 + 4)$ is an example of the

   (A) associative law of addition.
   (B) commutative law of multiplication.
   (C) associative law of multiplication.
   (D) commutative law of addition.

171. Evaluate the formula: $5x + 13y - 6z$, for $x = 2$, $y = 3$, and $z = 4$.

   (A) 25
   (B) 73
   (C) -5
   (D) -34

172. Evaluate the formula: $\dfrac{12+\left[15x-7y+2\right]}{8}$, for $x = 2$ and $y = 8$.

   (A) -3
   (B) 22
   (C) -11
   (D) 9

173. Evaluate the formula: $\dfrac{KL^2}{C}$, for $K = 5$, $L = 10$, and $C = 2$.

   (A) 1,000
   (B) 250
   (C) 25
   (D) 50

174. The volume of a cylinder is obtained as the product of π, its height (h) and its radius (r) squared. The corresponding formula is:

   (A) $\pi r \left(r^2 + h^2\right)^{\frac{1}{2}}$
   (B) $\pi r^2 h$
   (C) $2\pi rh$
   (D) πrh^2

175. Solve the following equation for x:
   $4x - 3 = -6x +17$.

   (A) 10
   (B) 7
   (C) 12
   (D) 2

176. Solve the following equation for *y*:

$$\frac{(2y+3)}{5} - 10 = \frac{(4-3y)}{2}.$$

- **(A)** 114
- **(B)** 24
- **(C)** 6
- **(D)** 9

177. Solve the following equation for *z*: $z + 5 = 4(z + 2) - (2z + 1)$.

- **(A)** 7
- **(B)** -2
- **(C)** 3
- **(D)** 2

178. If A is 4 times B and their sum is 30, what is the value of A?

- **(A)** 6
- **(B)** 12
- **(C)** 16
- **(D)** 24

179. John is now three times older than Harry is. Four years ago, John was five times as old as Harry was then. How old is John now?

- **(A)** 6 years old
- **(B)** 12 years old
- **(C)** 16 years old
- **(D)** 24 years old

180. Doug drove at a certain fixed speed for 2 hours. He then drove 20 miles per hour faster for 4 hours. The total distance covered was 320 miles. What speed, in miles per hour, did Doug maintain in the first leg of the trip?

- **(A)** 20 mph.
- **(B)** 30 mph.
- **(C)** 40 mph.
- **(D)** 50 mph.

181. Solve for *Y*: $5Y^2 = 10Y$. One solution is

- **(A)** 2
- **(B)** 5
- **(C)** 10
- **(D)** -5

182. Solve for *Z*: $aZ - b = cZ + d$.

- **(A)** $\dfrac{(d+b)}{(a-c)}$
- **(B)** $\dfrac{ac}{db}$
- **(C)** $\dfrac{(a-c)}{(d+b)}$
- **(D)** $\dfrac{(a-b)}{(c+d)}$

183. Solve for *A*: $8A - 17 > -7 + 3A$.

- **(A)** > 5
- **(B)** < 2
- **(C)** > -3
- **(D)** > 2

184. Solve for *B*: $\dfrac{B}{6} - \dfrac{B}{4} \geq 1$.

- **(A)** ≥ 6
- **(B)** ≤ -12
- **(C)** ≥ 12
- **(D)** ≤ 6

185. Solve for *C*: $3C - 18 < 8C - 3$.

- **(A)** < 6
- **(B)** < 8
- **(C)** > -3
- **(D)** < 3

GO ON TO THE NEXT PAGE

186. Solve for Y: $Y^2 + 7Y + 10 = 0$. One of the roots is

(A) 5

(B) -2

(C) 7

(D) -4

187. Solve for x: $x(x - 12) = 0$. One of the roots is

(A) -12

(B) 6

(C) 12

(D) -4

188. Solve for K: $K^2 + 36 = 5K^2$. One of the solutions is

(A) -3

(B) 6

(C) 4

(D) 12

189. Solve the simultaneous equations for C: $B + 2C = 12$ and $-B + 4C = 0$.

(A) 3

(B) -3

(C) 6

(D) 2

190. Solve the simultaneous equations for B: $2A + B = -7$ and $A - B = 1$.

(A) -3

(B) 7

(C) -4

(D) 6

191. Solve the simultaneous equations for R: $3R + 2S = 11$ and $5R - 4S = 22$.

(A) 11

(B) 4

(C) 3

(D) 7

192. If a patient is to take 2 tablets every morning and 1 tablet every evening, how many tablets will be required for a 14-day supply?

(A) 28

(B) 14

(C) 36

(D) 42

193. A formula for preparation of 200 milliliters of a lotion calls for 16 grams of calamine. How much calamine would be required to make 50 milliliters of the lotion?

(A) 32 grams

(B) 8 grams

(C) 4 grams

(D) 12 grams

194. How many grams of coal tar should be added to 450 grams of zinc oxide paste to prepare an ointment containing 10 percent coal tar?

(A) 50 grams

(B) 45 grams

(C) 90 grams

(D) 10 grams

195. A class of 5 students received test scores of 90, 80, 70, 80, and 90. What is their average score?

(A) 90

(B) 88

(C) 82

(D) 78

196. What is the median test score in the set of scores: 98, 62, 77, 96, 86, 93, and 72?

(A) 83

(B) 86

(C) 90

(D) 77

197. In triangle ABC, $AC = BC$. If the angle C is 30°, what is the angle A?

(A) 75°

(B) 45°

(C) 60°

(D) 30°

198. What is the length of the diagonal of a rectangle whose sides are 6 cm. and 8 cm. in length?

(A) 6 cm.

(B) 8 cm.

(C) 10 cm.

(D) 12 cm.

199. What is the area of a circle inscribed in a square whose sides are of length 8 inches?

(A) 64 sq. in.

(B) 50.2 sq. in.

(C) 38.6 sq. in.

(D) 24.2 sq. in.

200. Below, lines A and B are parallel. How many degrees is the angle α formed by lines B and C?

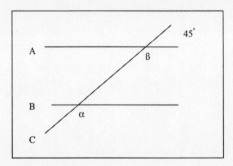

(A) 45°

(B) 150°

(C) 90°

(D) 135°

201. Label the sides of a rectangle A and B. Let B be 4 times greater than A. If the area of the rectangle is 100, what is the value of B?

(A) 5

(B) 10

(C) 15

(D) 20

202. What is the area of a square inscribed in a circle of diameter 10?

(A) 100

(B) 50

(C) 80

(D) 200

203. The x- and y-coordinates of a point can be represented as (x, y). What is the distance between the two points $(-3, 2)$ and $(1, -1)$?

(A) 5

(B) 12

(C) 7

(D) 3.2

204. If the perimeter of a triangle ABC is 270, with $AB = 35$ and $AC = 150$, what is BC?

(A) 125

(B) 70

(C) 55

(D) 85

205. If the volume of a cube is 1,000 cubic inches, what is its surface area?

(A) 100 sq. in.

(B) 500 sq. in.

(C) 600 sq. in.

(D) 2,000 sq. in.

GO ON TO THE NEXT PAGE

206. If a line is represented by the equation $Y = 5x + 25$, what is its x-intercept?

(A) 25

(B) -10

(C) -5

(D) 15

207. What is the equation for the straight line in the XY plot below?

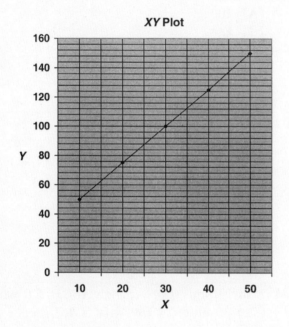

XY Plot

(A) $Y = 2.5x + 25$

(B) $Y = 10x + 50$

(C) $Y = 25x - 10$

(D) $Y = 12.5x + 5$

Question 208 uses the graph below.

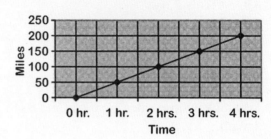

Driving Speed

208. What is the slope of the straight line in the graph?

(A) 10

(B) 25

(C) 50

(D) 75

Question 209 uses the graph below.

Distribution of Household Pets in Amite City

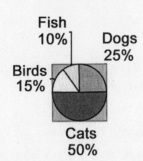

Fish 10%

Dogs 25%

Birds 15%

Cats 50%

209. If there are 5,000 dogs in Amite City, how many pet birds are there?

(A) 750

(B) 2,000

(C) 3,000

(D) 10,000

Question 210 uses the graph below.

Yearly U.S. Spending on Magnetic Fusion Energy

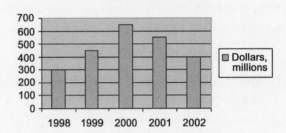

Dollars, millions

210. How much less was spent on magnetic fusion energy in the year 2002 than in 2000?

(A) $100 million

(B) $150 million

(C) $250 million

(D) $300 million

S T O P If you finish before time is called, you may check your work on this section only. Do not turn to any other section in the test.

CHEMISTRY

Number of Questions: 60
Time: 30 MINUTES

Directions: For questions 211–270, select the correct answer and mark it on your answer sheet. There is only one correct answer for each question.

211. The binding strength (concentration at IC50) of a potential drug to its receptor is usually expressed in nM. A concentration of 1 nM is equal to

  (A) 10^{-3}M.

  (B) 10^{-6}M.

  (C) 10^{-9}M.

  (D) 10^{-12}M.

212. How much sodium hydroxide (Na = 23, O = 16, H = 1) is needed to make a 500ml. of 0.3M solution of sodium hydroxide?

  (A) 20 g.

  (B) 12 g.

  (C) 9 g.

  (D) 6 g.

213. A student mixes a 500ml. of 1M sodium chloride solution with a 200ml. of 2M sodium chloride solution, then adds water to make the final volume 2,000 ml. The final concentration of sodium chloride is

  (A) 0.9M.

  (B) 0.45M.

  (C) 0.25M.

  (D) 0.2M.

214. Solution A has a pH = 9, and solution B has a pH = 5, therefore

  (A) both A and B are acidic.

  (B) both A and B are basic.

  (C) A is basic and B is acidic.

  (D) A is acidic and B is basic.

215. With regard to significant figures, the correct result of 10.3 + 1.52 + 3.014 should be

  (A) 14.8

  (B) 14.83

  (C) 14.834

  (D) 15

216. Oxygen-17 has 8 protons and 9 neutrons. How many electrons does it have?

  (A) 16 electrons

  (B) 9 electrons

  (C) 17 electrons

  (D) 8 electrons

217. Which of the following statement about isotopes is false?

  (A) They have the same valence.

  (B) They have the same number of electrons.

  (C) They have the same mass.

  (D) They have the same chemical property.

218. Name the hydrocarbon $CH_3(CH_2)_5CH_3$.

(A) Heptane

(B) Pentane

(C) Octane

(D) Decane

219. Which of the following statements about ethylene is false?

(A) Atoms in double bonds are not free to rotate.

(B) The bond length between the carbons is shorter than in ethane.

(C) The carbon has a *sp* hybrid orbital.

(D) It is a symmetric molecule.

220. CH_3- group is called the

(A) methyl group.

(B) methylene group.

(C) methane group.

(D) methine group.

221. Which symbols can be used to assign the absolute configuration of a chiral molecule?

(A) E and Z

(B) Syn and anti

(C) Cis and trans

(D) R and S

222. With regard to hybrid orbitals, which statement is true about the oxygen in water and the nitrogen in ammonia?

(A) Both have *sp*

(B) Both have *sp²*

(C) Both have *sp³*

(D) Water has *sp²* and ammonia has *sp³*

223. The percent composition by mass of a compound is important to verify the purity of a compound. What is the percentage composition by mass of hydrogen in H_2O_2 (H = 1, and O = 16)?

(A) 2 percent

(B) 5.9 percent

(C) 6.2 percent

(D) 50 percent

224. The correct name for HOCl is

(A) hypochlorous acid.

(B) chlorous acid.

(C) chloric acid.

(D) perchloric acid.

225. The balanced equation for $KClO_3 ==> KCl + O_2$ is

(A) $KClO_3 ==> KCl + 3O_2$.

(B) $2KClO_3 ==> 2KCl + O_2$.

(C) $2KClO_3 ==> KCl + 3O_2$.

(D) $2KClO_3 ==> 2KCl + 3O_2$.

226. Which compound is classified as a weak electrolyte in solution?

(A) Sodium hydroxide

(B) Acetic acid

(C) Hydrochloric acid

(D) Sodium carbonate

227. By definition of Brønsted theory, $H_2PO_4^-$ is a(n)

(A) acid only.

(B) base only.

(C) acid and a base.

(D) None of the above

GO ON TO THE NEXT PAGE

228. In the reaction of $2Ca(s) + O_2(g) \rightarrow 2CaO(s)$, which statement is false?

(A) The calcium atom loses electrons.

(B) The oxygen atom loses electrons.

(C) The entropy decreases in the reaction.

(D) Calcium is a reducing agent.

229. At 1 atm and 0°C, 1 gram of hydrogen gas occupies a volume of (atomic weight of H = 1)?

(A) 11.2 liters

(B) 22.4 liters

(C) 1 liter

(D) 760 liters

230. Under the same temperature and pressure, which statement is true about the effusion rates of nitrogen and oxygen molecules in gas state (atomic weight: O = 16 and N = 14)?

(A) Nitrogen is faster.

(B) Oxygen is faster.

(C) The rates are the same.

(D) It cannot be determined.

231. The maximum number of electrons present in the principle level for which n = 2 is

(A) 2

(B) 4

(C) 6

(D) 8

232. The exclusion principle, which states that no two electrons in an atom can have the same four quantum numbers, is associated with

(A) Heisenberg.

(B) Pauli.

(C) Bohr.

(D) Planck.

233. Which simple molecule does NOT have a planar geometry?

(A) Benzene

(B) BF_3

(C) NH_3

(D) Ethylene

234. Which molecule does NOT have a pi bond?

(A) Methanol

(B) Formaldehyde

(C) Acetone

(D) Naphthalene

235. Which atoms are least likely to form hydrogen bonding?

(A) Fluorine

(B) Nitrogen

(C) Oxygen

(D) Carbon

236. Acetic acid is soluble in nonpolar solvent such as benzene, because acetic acid

(A) is a nonpolar molecule.

(B) is an aromatic compound.

(C) can react with benzene.

(D) molecules can form Dimmer's.

237. In the *homolysis* process, red blood cells are placed in a water solution in which the cells swell and eventually burst. This process is based on the phenomena of osmosis. The water solution in this process is considered to be a(n)

(A) isotonic solution.

(B) hypertonic solution.

(C) hypotonic solution.

(D) osmotic solution.

238. In reference to ion-product constant for water K_w, which statement is false?

   (A) $K_w = [H^+][OH^-]$.

   (B) K_w is temperature dependent.

   (C) K_w does not depend on pH.

   (D) K_w is pressure dependent.

239. At 25°C, the $[OH^-]$ concentration of a solution with pH = 4 is

   (A) 10^{-12}M.

   (B) 10^{-10}M.

   (C) 10^{-7}M.

   (D) 10^{-4}M.

240. Pick out the false statement about acid and base.

   (A) The stronger the acid, the stronger its conjugate base.

   (B) Strong acids are strong electrolytes.

   (C) NH_4^+ is the conjugate acid of NH_3.

   (D) H_3O^+ is the strongest acid that can exist in aqueous solution.

241. Which acid is the strongest?

   (A) Hypochlorous acid

   (B) Chlorous acid

   (C) Chloric acid

   (D) Perchloric acid

242. Oxides can be classified as acidic, basic, and amphoteric based on their reaction with water. Which of the following oxides is NOT an acidic oxide?

   (A) CO_2

   (B) As_2O_3

   (C) CaO

   (D) SO_2

243. For a 0.1M solution of weak acid HA, which is true?

   (A) pH = 1

   (B) pH > 1

   (C) pH < 1

   (D) It cannot be determined.

244. Considering $K_a = 4.9 \times 10^{-10}$ for HCN and $K_b = 1.8 \times 10^{-5}$ for NH_3, which statement about NH_4CN is true? (Hint: No calculation is necessary.)

   (A) The solution is basic.

   (B) The solution is acidic.

   (C) The solution is neutral.

   (D) It cannot be determined.

245. Which of the following solutions is NOT a buffer system?

   (A) CH_3COONa/CH_3COOH

   (B) $KClO_4/HClO_4$

   (C) KH_2PO_4/H_3PO_4

   (D) NH_3/NH_4NO_3

246. When 18 g. of water vapor condenses to 18 g. of water, the entropy

   (A) equals to 1mol.

   (B) does not change.

   (C) increases.

   (D) decreases.

247. Mercury (Hg) is the only metal that exists as a liquid at room temperature. The two oxidation states in which mercury exists are

   (A) divalent and tetravalent.

   (B) monovalent and divalent.

   (C) monovalent and trivalent.

   (D) divalent and trivalent.

GO ON TO THE NEXT PAGE

248. With regard to halogens, which of the following statement is false?

(A) Atomic radius increases as F < Cl < Br < I.

(B) Acid strength of hydrogen halides increases as HF < HCl < HBr <HI.

(C) All halogens form diatomic molecules in their elemental state.

(D) All halogens can have oxidation number of +7 in their compounds.

249. All of the following are properties of hydrogen peroxide EXCEPT it

(A) is a planar molecule in geometry.

(B) can act as an oxidation agent.

(C) can act as a reducing agent.

(D) is easily miscible with water.

250. The decay of carbon isotope ^{14}C is used to determine the ages of certain objects. The ^{14}C isotope (atomic mass = 14, atomic number = 6) decays to ^{14}N (atomic mass = 14, atomic number = 7) with an emission of a particle. This particle is mostly likely a(n)

(A) proton.

(B) neutron.

(C) electron.

(D) α particle.

251. Which of the following statements about rotation around the chemical bond is false?

(A) Atoms in double bonds are not free to rotate.

(B) Atoms in a ring are not free to rotate.

(C) Atoms in single bonds are free to rotate.

(D) Atoms in triple bonds are free to rotate.

252. The number of structural isomers that C_5H_{12} can have is

(A) 2

(B) 3

(C) 4

(D) 5

253. The two geometric isomers of dibromoehtylene, BrHC = CHBr, are called

(A) R- and s- isomers.

(B) O- and p- isomers.

(C) Cis- and trans- isomers.

(D) N- and t- isomers.

254. What functional group does molecule $CH_2OHCOCH=CHCHO$ NOT have?

(A) Ketone

(B) Hydroxyl

(C) Aldehyde

(D) Ester

255. If H_2SO_4 is sulfuric acid, which of the following choices is sulfurous acid?

(A) H_2SO_3

(B) H_2S

(C) H_3SO_3

(D) H_3SO_4

256. In the reaction of $(CH_3)_2C=CH-CH_3 + HBr \rightarrow$ $(CH_3)_2CBr-CH_2CH_3$, the hydrogen from HBr goes to the CH instead of C in the double bond. This is known as

(A) Avogadro's law.

(B) Markovnikov's rule.

(C) Boyle's law.

(D) Saytzeff's rule.

257. In which compound does the carbon have the highest positive oxidation number?

(A) Carbon dioxide

(B) Methanol

(C) Formic acid

(D) Methane

258. The esterification reaction converts alcohol to esters. For the reaction, $CH_3COOH + CH_3CH_2OH \rightarrow CH_3COOCH_2CH_3 + H_2O$, which reactant(s) provide the –OH group?

(A) CH_3CH_2OH

(B) CH_3COOH

(C) Half of CH_3CH_2OH and half of CH_3COOH

(D) None of the above

259. In which order does the acidity increase for the following compounds?

(A) Methanol < acetic acid < phenol

(B) Acetic acid < methanol < phenol

(C) Phenol < methanol < acetic acid

(D) Methanol < phenol < acetic acid

260. The Tollen's test (silver-mirror test) will generally provide positive results for which group of compounds?

(A) Esters

(B) Amines

(C) Ketones

(D) Aldehyde

261. For a compound with three non-identical asymmetric carbon atoms, the maximum number of possible stereoisomers is

(A) 3

(B) 6

(C) 8

(D) 9

262. Glucose is the key sugar of the body and known as the "blood sugar." Which is NOT a property of this compound?

(A) It is optically active.

(B) It is sweeter than sucrose.

(C) It gives positive results for Tollen's test.

(D) It can be reduced by H_2/Pt to a polyhydroxy alcohol.

263. Which amino acid is most likely to be classified as neutral amino acid?

(A) Glycine

(B) Lysine

(C) Arginine

(D) Histidine

264. Amides may have all of the following formulas EXCEPT

(A) $R-CO-NH_2$.

(B) $R-CO-NHR$.

(C) $R-CO-NR_3$.

(D) $R-CO-NR_2$.

265. How many isomers does trichlorobenzene have?

(A) 2

(B) 3

(C) 4

(D) 5

266. In organic chemistry, the Diels-Alder reaction involves a(n)

(A) carboxylic acid and an alcohol.

(B) alkene and a halogen.

(C) acid and a base.

(D) alkene and a diene.

GO ON TO THE NEXT PAGE

267. What is the general formula for esters?

    (A) RCOOR'

    (B) ROR'

    (C) RCOR'

    (D) ROH

268. Lipids are the major components of cell membranes. Which of the following compounds can NOT be classified as a lipid?

    (A) Fatty acids

    (B) Steroids

    (C) Starch

    (D) Cholesterol

269. A primary amines has at least 2 hydrogens attached to the nitrogen atom. A tertiary amine has

    (A) no hydrogen attached to the nitrogen atom.

    (B) only 1 hydrogen attached to the nitrogen atom.

    (C) 2 hydrogens attached to the nitrogen atom.

    (D) 3 hydrogens attached to the nitrogen atom.

270. In proteins, the α-helix and β-sheet refer to what level of protein structure?

    (A) Primary structure

    (B) Secondary structure

    (C) Tertiary structure

    (D) All of the above

STOP   If you finish before time is called, you may check your work on this section only. Do not turn to any other section in the test.

ANSWER KEY

Reading Composition

1. B	10. B	19. D	28. A	37. A
2. C	11. B	20. B	29. B	38. B
3. D	12. B	21. A	30. D	39. D
4. A	13. C	22. D	31. C	40. A
5. C	14. B	23. B	32. D	41. D
6. B	15. C	24. A	33. A	42. B
7. A	16. B	25. C	34. B	43. C
8. D	17. D	26. B	35. D	44. B
9. C	18. C	27. D	36. A	45. D

Verbal Ability

46. D	56. D	66. D	76. A	86. D
47. B	57. A	67. B	77. B	87. D
48. B	58. A	68. C	78. A	88. A
49. A	59. A	69. A	79. C	89. B
50. C	60. A	70. C	80. A	90. C
51. D	61. A	71. A	81. D	91. D
52. B	62. D	72. D	82. A	92. A
53. A	63. A	73. C	83. A	93. A
54. B	64. D	74. A	84. B	94. B
55. A	65. C	75. D	85. A	95. A

Biology

96. C	106. B	116. B	126. B	136. D
97. A	107. B	117. C	127. A	137. B
98. B	108. A	118. C	128. D	138. B
99. B	109. B	119. D	129. D	139. B
100. A	110. D	120. D	130. C	140. D
101. D	111. D	121. C	131. B	141. C
102. D	112. C	122. C	132. B	142. D
103. A	113. A	123. B	133. A	143. B
104. A	114. B	124. D	134. C	144. B
105. C	115. B	125. A	135. B	145. C

Quantitative Ability

146. C	159. D	172. D	185. C	198. C
147. A	160. A	173. B	186. B	199. B
148. B	161. B	174. B	187. C	200. D
149. C	162. D	175. D	188. A	201. D
150. A	163. D	176. C	189. D	202. B
151. D	164. C	177. B	190. A	203. A
152. B	165. B	178. D	191. B	204. D
153. A	166. D	179. D	192. D	205. C
154. D	167. D	180. C	193. C	206. C
155. B	168. B	181. A	194. A	207. A
156. B	169. A	182. A	195. C	208. C
157. C	170. C	183. D	196. B	209. C
158. A	171. A	184. B	197. A	210. C

Chemistry

211. C	223. B	235. D	247. B	259. D
212. D	224. A	236. D	248. D	260. D
213. B	225. D	237. C	249. A	261. C
214. C	226. B	238. D	250. C	262. B
215. A	227. C	239. B	251. D	263. A
216. D	228. B	240. A	252. B	264. C
217. C	229. A	241. D	253. C	265. B
218. A	230. A	242. C	254. D	266. D
219. C	231. D	243. B	255. A	267. A
220. A	232. B	244. A	256. B	268. C
221. D	233. C	245. B	257. A	269. A
222. C	234. A	246. D	258. B	270. B

EXPLANATORY ANSWERS

Reading Comprehension

1. **The correct answer is (B).** The answer to the question is found in **lines 26–27** of the paragraph: "Three problems lead to esophageal dysphagia: impaired esophageal peristaltic motility, esophageal obstruction, and acid reflux . . . ."

2. **The correct answer is (C).** The answer to the question is found in **line 10** of the paragraph: "The average esophagus is about 9 to 10 inches long . . . . "

3. **The correct answer is (D).** The answer to the question is found in **lines 1–2** of the paragraph: "Fifty pairs of muscles . . . ."

4. **The correct answer is (A).** The answer to the question is found in **lines 6–7** of the paragraph: ". . . the pharynx, the canal that connects the mouth to the . . . ."

5. **The correct answer is (C).** The answer to the question is found in **line 19** of the paragraph: "The vast majority of disorders occur in the involuntary state 2 (oropharyngeal dysphagia) and stage 3 . . . ."

6. **The correct answer is (B).** The answer to the question is found in **lines 24 and 25** of the paragraph: "Oropharyngeal dysphagia is the most common subtype observed among the elderly, ..."

7. **The correct answer is (A).** The answer to the question is found in **line 11** of the paragraph: ". . . through the upper esophageal sphincter, a one-way valve . . . ."

8. **The correct answer is (D).** The answer to the question is found in **line 8** of the paragraph: "The larynx, meanwhile, closes tightly . . . ."

9. **The correct answer is (C).** The answer to the question is found in **line 14** of the paragraph: "Injectable botulinum toxin type B solution (Myobloc, ... "

10. **The correct answer is (B).** The answer to the question is found in **lines 6 and 7** of the paragraph: "Botulinum toxin type B, a neurotoxin produced by Clostridium botulinum, acts by blocking acetylcholine release at the neuromuscular junction."

11. **The correct answer is (B).** The answer to the question is found in **lines 7 and 8** of the paragraph: "Botulinum toxin type B, unlike botulinum toxin type A, is available as a sterile solution for injection . . . ."

12. **The correct answer is (B).** The answer to the question is found in **line 1** of the paragraph: "Headache is the most common patient complaint reported . . . ."

13. **The correct answer is (C).** The answer to the question is found in **lines 8–10** of the paragraph: "Because of differences in vehicles, dilution schemes, and laboratory protocols for determining the median lethal dose in mice, units of biological activity of botulinum toxin type B cannot be . . . ."

14. **The correct answer is (B).** The answer to the question is found in **lines 16 and 17** of the paragraph: "The severity of headaches was recorded by the patient on a scale from 0-5, where 0 = no headache and 5 = severe headache. . . ."

15. **The correct answer is (C).** The answer to the question is found in **lines 2 and 3** of the paragraph: "...whether primary headaches (such as tension headache, migraine headache, cluster headache, and rebound headache ...."

16. **The correct answer is (B).** The answer to the question is found in **line 18** of the paragraph: "Botulinum toxin type B was given every three ...."

17. **The correct answer is (D).** The answer to the question is found in **lines 11 and 12** of the paragraph: "However, botulinum toxin type B 5,000 units/ml. is generally considered to have a therapeutic effect ...."

18. **The correct answer is (C).** The answer to the question is found in **line 14** of the paragraph: "... was used at a neurology clinic ...."

19. **The correct answer is (D).** The answer to the question is found in **line 11** of the paragraph: "The first paper, Tuschl explains, 'is the ....'"

20. **The correct answer is (B).** The answer to the question is found in **line 8** of the paragraph: "... engineered small inhibitory RNAs (siRNAs) ...."

21. **The correct answer is (A).** The answer to the question is found in **line 2** of the paragraph: "After Fire and colleagues first reported ...."

22. **The correct answer is (D).** The answer to the question is found in **line 18** of the paragraph: "But Tuschl's group, using a *Drosopbila* lysate system ...."

23. **The correct answer is (B).** The answer to the question is found in **line 22** of the paragraph: "Identifying the siRNA lengths that best ...."

24. **The correct answer is (A).** The answer to the question is found in **line 13** of the paragraph: "... occurring system, posttranscriptional gene silencing (PTGS) ...."

25. **The correct answer is (C).** The answer to the question is found in **lines 27 and 28** of the paragraph: "The key to inhibition of mammalian gene ...."

26. **The correct answer is (B).** The answer to the question is found in **line 12** of the paragraph: "... shows that siRNAs can direct gene ...."

27. **The correct answer is (D).** The answer to the question is found in **line 19** of the paragraph: ".... occurs when the RNA fragments are 21- or 22-nucleotide duplexes of sense and antisense RNA."

28. **The correct answer is (A).** The answer to the question is found in **line 30** of the paragraph: "'Once we showed how it worked in flies ... we could go into mammalian cells and see if we....'"

29. **The correct answer is (B).** The answer to the question is found in **line 30** of the paragraph: "Once we showed how it worked in flies ...."

30. **The correct answer is (D).** The answer to the question is found in **line 33** of the paragraph: "This paper showed that ... an intermediate in the RNAi pathway (siRNA), could be successfully used to initiate ...."

31. **The correct answer is (C).** The answer to the question is found in **line 2** of the paragraph: "... would typically take 20 person-years to produce...."

32. **The correct answer is (D).** The answer to the question is found in **line 8** of the paragraph: "Other bottlenecks include data collection and data analysis."

33. **The correct answer is (A).** The answer to the question is found in **line 22** of the paragraph: "... says that crystallization was, is, and will be a rate-limiting step."

34. **The correct answer is (B).** The answer to the question is found in **lines 9 and 10** of the paragraph: "...high-throughput (HT) methods ...."

35. **The correct answer is (D).** The answer to the question is found in **lines 17 and 18** of the paragraph: "... structure once every decade to solving 75 percent ...."

36. **The correct answer is (A).** The answer to the question is found in **lines 4 and 5** of the paragraph: "... obtaining a suitable crystal."

37. **The correct answer is (A).** The answer to the question is found in **lines 13 and 14** of the paragraph: "... and ultimately, for translating raw genomic information into new pharmaceuticals."

38. **The correct answer is (B).** The answer to the question is found in **line 15** of the paragraph: "The conductances of gated channels such as MscS ...."

39. **The correct answer is (D).** The answer to the question is found in **line 1** of the paragraph: "The mechanosensitive channel of small conductance, MscS, was ...."

40. **The correct answer is (A).** The answer to the question is found in **lines 2 and 3** of the paragraph: "... conductance of ~1 nS, with a slight preference for anions ...."

41. **The correct answer is (D).** The answer to the question is found in **lines 23 and 24** of the paragraph: "... to date, no structure of a voltage-gated system ...."

42. **The correct answer is (B).** The answer to the question is found in **line 5** of the paragraph: "Both MscS and MscL are intrinsically mechanosensitive, ..."

43. **The correct answer is (C).** The answer to the question is found in **lines 21 and 22** of the paragraph: "... a prokaryotic potassium channel by proton binding to the channel and by calcium binding to an extramembrane domain."

44. **The correct answer is (B).** The answer to the question is found in **line 11** of the paragraph: "... the *E. coli* protein, with 286 amino acids is predicted ...."

45. **The correct answer is (D).** The answer to the question is found in **line 7** of the paragraph: "... threshold for MscS opening is ~ 50 percent that of MscL, ..."

Verbal Ability

46. The correct answer is (D).

EXISTENCE (n.)—the fact or state of existing or being. *Nonexistence* (n.)—the condition of not existing.

47. The correct answer is (B).

KNOWABLE (adj.)—having a direct cognition or understanding of. *Unknowable* (adj.)—impossible to know or understand.

48. The correct answer is (B).

INTERFUSION (n.)—combination caused by fusing or blending. *Splitting* (v.)—separating or dividing into parts.

49. The correct answer is (A).

INTIMATE (n.)—close friend or confidant. *Stranger* (n.)—a foreigner or newcomer.

50. The correct answer is (C).

METAMORPHOSE (v.)—to change or transform into a different appearance. *Static* (adj.)—fixed or stationary.

51. The correct answer is (D).

OUTCRY (n.)—a loud cry or clamor. *Acquiescence* (n.)—passive assent or agreement without protest.

52. The correct answer is (B).

RUBBISH (n.)—something that is worthless or nonsensical. *Factual* (adj.)—of or containing facts.

53. The correct answer is (A).

SHANTY (n.)—a small, roughly built dwelling or shelter. *Estate* (n.)—a landed property, usually with a large house on it.

54. The correct answer is (B).

ABDICATION (n.)—the act or state of relinquishing power or responsibility. *Enlistment* (n.)—active participation in a cause or enterprise.

55. The correct answer is (A).

ASCRIBE (v.)—to refer to a supposed cause, source, or author. *Abstain* (v.)—to refrain from something by one's own choice.

56. The correct answer is (D).

CREDIBLE (adj.)—offering reasonable grounds for being believed. *Distrust* (n.)—lack of trust or confidence.

57. The correct answer is (A).

PERENNIALLY (adv.)—active through the year or many years. *Annually* (adv.)—recurring or performed every year.

58. The correct answer is (A).

EMINENCE (n.)—a position of prominence or superiority. *Level* (n.)—a position in scale or rank.

59. The correct answer is (A).

TANGLE (v.)—to involve, as to hamper or obstruct. *Untangle* (v.)—to loose from tangles.

60. The correct answer is (A).

CAVILING (v.)—raising irritating and trivial objections. *Appreciative* (adj.)—having or showing appreciation.

61. The correct answer is (A).

DECLINATION (n.)—the action or process of deteriorating or declining. *Ascension* (n.)—the process of moving or sloping upward.

62. The correct answer is (D).

EMANATE (v.)—to come out from a source. *Rescind* (v.)—to take away or remove.

63. The correct answer is (A).

DEFENSIBLE (adj.)—capable of being defended. *Indefensible* (adj.)—incapable of being maintained as right or valid; incapable of being protected.

64. The correct answer is (D).

EMPIRICAL (adj.)—based on observation or experience. *Absolute* (adj.)—free from imperfection; complete.

65. The correct answer is (C).

EYEWASH (n.)—misleading or deceptive statements, actions, or procedures. *Truth* (n.)—the property of being in accord with fact or reality.

66. The correct answer is (D).

PURPOSELESS (adj.)—lacking a purpose; meaningless or aimless. *Directed* (adj.)—proceeding without interruption in a straight course or line.

67. The correct answer is (B).

GENIALITY (n.)—an act marked by kindness and courtesy. *Rudeness* (adj.)—lacking the graces and refinement of civilized life.

68. The correct answer is (C).

HARNESS (v.)—to bring under control and direct the force of. *Unprotected* (adj.)—not protected; open to assault, injury, damage, or theft.

69. The correct answer is (A).

HYPOTHESIS (n.)—an assumption or concession made for the sake of argument. *Fact* (n.)—knowledge or information based on real occurrences.

70. **The correct answer is (C).**

IMPONDERABLE (adj.)— incapable of being weighed or evaluated with exactness. *Ponderable* (adj.)—significant enough to be worth considering.

71. **The correct answer is (A).**

APPLAUDING (v.)—expressing approval of or praising. *Adulating* (v.)—praising or admiring excessively.

72. **The correct answer is (D).**

DIVORCE (n.)—the action or an instance of legally dissolving a marriage. *Sunder* (v.)—to break or wrench apart; sever.

73. **The correct answer is (C).**

PHARMACIST (n.)—a person trained in pharmacy. *Apothecary* (n.)—one who prepares and sells drugs or compounds for medicinal purposes.

74. **The correct answer is (A).**

DOCK (n.)—the area of water between two piers or alongside a pier that receives a ship for loading, unloading, or repairs. *Pier* (n.)—a platform extending from a shore over water and supported by piles or pillars.

75. **The correct answer is (D).**

RESULT (n.)—the consequence of a particular action. *Sequence* (n.)—a following of one thing after another.

76. **The correct answer is (A).**

FERTILE (adj.)—capable of initiating, sustaining, or supporting reproduction. *Fecund* (adj.)—capable of producing offspring or vegetation.

77. **The correct answer is (B).**

AUBERGE (n.)—an establishment for the lodging and entertaining of travelers. *Caravansary* (n.)—an inn surrounding a court in eastern countries where caravans of people rest at night.

78. **The correct answer is (A).**

DEAN (n.)—the head of a division, faculty, college, or school of a university. *Leader* (n.)—one who leads or guides.

79. **The correct answer is (C).**

ENGAGING (adv.)—holding the attention of. *Loathsome* (adj.)—offensive or disgusting.

80. **The correct answer is (A).**

WALLFLOWER (n.)—one who does not participate in the activity at a social event because of shyness or unpopularity. *Dancer* (n.)—a person engaged in or performing a dance.

81. The correct answer is (D).

JOHN DORY (n.)—a North Atlantic fish with a laterally compressed body and long spines on the dorsal fin. *Fish* (n.)—an aquatic animal.

82. The correct answer is (A).

MENIAL (n.)—a person doing menial work, specifically a domestic servant. *Dray horse* (n.)—a horse adapted for drawing heavy loads.

83. The correct answer is (A).

AGREEMENT (n.)—harmony of opinion or accord. *Contract* (n.)—the writing or document containing an agreement.

84. The correct answer is (B).

VORTEX (n.)—a spiral motion of fluid within a limited area. *Maelstrom* (n.)—a whirlpool of extraordinary size or violence.

85. The correct answer is (A).

WAGGLE (v.)—to move frequently one way and the other. *Switch* (v.)—a shift from one to another.

86. The correct answer is (D).

LIAR (n.)—one that tells lies. *Perjurer* (n.)—a person who deliberately gives false testimony.

87. The correct answer is (D).

TACKY (adj.)—lacking style or good taste. *Modish* (adj.)—fashionable or stylish.

88. The correct answer is (A).

WRECKAGE (n.)—the act of wrecking or the state of being wrecked. *Sabotage* (n.)—destruction of property or obstruction of normal operations.

89. The correct answer is (B).

THESPIAN (n.)—an actor or actress. *Mummer* (n.)—a performer or actor in a pantomime.

90. The correct answer is (C).

ANNIHILATE (v.)—to destroy completely. *Invent* (v.)—to produce or contrive by the use of ingenuity or imagination.

91. The correct answer is (D).

HARE (n.)—any of various swift long-eared lagomorph mammals. *Slowpoke* (n.)—one that moves, works, or acts slowly.

92. The correct answer is (A).

RECREANT (adj.)—unfaithful or disloyal to a belief, duty, or cause. *Perfidious* (adj.)—of, relating to, or marked by perfidy; treacherous.

93. **The correct answer is (A).**

POLITY (n.)—the form of government of a nation, state, church, or organization. *Course* (n.)—the act or action of moving in a path from point to point.

94. **The correct answer is (B).**

IRASCIBLE (adj.)—marked by hot temper and easily provoked anger. *Tolerant* (adj.)—inclined to bear or put up with.

95. **The correct answer is (A).**

HORRID (adj.)—causing horror; dreadful. *Lurid* (adj.)—causing shock or horror; gruesome.

Biology

96. **The correct answer is (C).** Exocrine glands include merocrine, halocrine, and apocrine glands.

97. **The correct answer is (A).** According to the Fluid Mosaic Model, the cell membrane consists of a bilayer of phospholipid molecules with the *inner* membrane being hydrophilic and the *exterior* surface being hydrophobic.

98. **The correct answer is (B).** Facilitated diffusion is similar to simple diffusion except that carrier proteins are required for transport of molecules.

99. **The correct answer is (B).** *Pacinian* corpuscles are located in deep dermis and subcutaneous regions. *Meissner's* corpuscles are located in dermal papillae.

100. **The correct answer is (A).** Stimulation of Ca^{++} resorption in the kidney tubules is a function of the parathyroid hormone, which is secreted by the parathyroid gland.

101. **The correct answer is (D).** The *epiphyseal growth plate* is the portion of the epiphyses where active proliferation of cartilage takes place.

102. **The correct answer is (D).** Muscle contraction involves the interaction between actin and myosin. This interaction is facilitated by the presence of calcium and ATP.

103. **The correct answer is (A).** Acetylcholine (ACh) is released from a motor end fiber, causing stimulation of the sarcolemma of muscle fiber.

104. **The correct answer is (A).** *Glycolysis* is the aerobic conversion of a 6-carbon sugar (e.g., glucose) to two pyruvate molecules resulting in the formation of 38 ATP molecules from a single glucose molecule. *Anaerobic glycolysis* results in alcohol and lactic acid fermentation.

105. **The correct answer is (C).** *Myelin* is produced by oligodendrocytes in the central nervous system and Schwann cells in the peripheral nervous system.

106. **The correct answer is (B).** Na^+ is in high concentration outside the cell.

107. **The correct answer is (B).** The synapse is a specialized junction between 2 neurons where the impulse is transferred from the presynaptic neuron to the postsynaptic neuron.

108. **The correct answer is (A).** Neurotransmitter clearance from the synaptic cleft can occur via degradation by specific enzymes (e.g., acetylcholine is destroyed by acetylcholinesterase) or reuptake into storage vesicles within the presynaptic membrane.

109. **The correct answer is (B).** Nociceptors do not undergo sensory adaptation, which is a phenomenon where stimulus response diminishes with constant stimulation.

110. **The correct answer is (D).** *Lipitor* is commonly used to lower cholesterol.

111. **The correct answer is (D).** Sense of taste is relayed via two pathways. The anterior $\frac{2}{3}$ of the tongue is associated with CN VII and the posterior $\frac{1}{3}$ of the tongue is associated with CN IX.

112. **The correct answer is (C).** *Sebaceous* glands are exocrine glands that secrete oil.

113. **The correct answer is (A).** *Anti-diruetic hormone* and *oxytocin* are secreted by the posterior pituitary gland. *Aldosterone* is secreted by the adrenal glands.

114. **The correct answer is (B).** The Islets of Langerhans are the endocrine glands of the pancreas. Insulin produced by the β-cells within the Islets of Langerhans functions to *decrease* blood glucose levels. Glucagon produced by the α-cells within the Islets of Langerhans functions to *increase* blood glucose levels.

115. **The correct answer is (B).** In general, arteries carry blood rich in oxygen and low in carbon dioxide. The reverse is true for arteries.

116. **The correct answer is (B).** The pulmonary and aortic semilunar valves lie within the pulmonary trunk and the aorta, respectively. The bicuspid valve separates the left atrium and ventricle.

117. **The correct answer is (C).** The *atrioventricular node* serves as a delay signal that allows for ventricular filling. *Purkinje fibers* conduct the impulse into the mass of ventricular muscle tissue. The *atrioventricular bundle* serves as an electrical connection between the atria and ventricles.

118. **The correct answer is (C).** The *T wave* represents ventricular repolarization. The *QRS complex* represents the onset of ventricular depolarization. The *P wave* represents atrial depolarization.

119. **The correct answer is (D).** Cardiac output is the product of heart rate and stroke volume.

120. **The correct answer is (D).** *Histamine* acts to decrease blood pressure.

121. **The correct answer is (C).** *T-cells* are specialized leukocytes that are involved in mediating the specific immune response.

122. **The correct answer is (C).** The *lymphatic system* is involved in transporting lipids and lipid-soluble vitamins absorbed in the gastrointestinal tract to the blood stream.

123. **The correct answer is (B).** T-cells undergo selection and maturation in the *thymus*.

124. **The correct answer is (D).** Antibodies are produced by B-cells, and serve as an integral component of the specific immune response.

125. **The correct answer is (A).** The *macrophage* engulfs the foreign particle and presents surface antigen that is recognized by T-cells. B-cells respond to activated T-cells by secreting antibodies.

126. **The correct answer is (B).** *IgA* molecules help defend against bacterial cells and viruses. *IgM* molecules are the first to be secreted after antigen exposure. *IgG* molecules defend against bacterial cells, viruses, and toxins.

127. **The correct answer is (A).** *Gastrin* is responsible for gastroesophageal sphincter contraction. *Lipases* found in pancreatic juice are responsible for the breakdown of fats and triglycerides. *Secretin* stimulates the release of pancreatic juice into the duodenum.

128. **The correct answer is (D).** The *gall bladder* is responsible for bile storage and concentration between meals.

129. **The correct answer is (D).** The majority of nutrient absorption takes place in the *small intestine*.

130. **The correct answer is (C).** *Vital capacity* is the maximum volume of air that a person can expire after maximal inspiration. *Inspiratory Reserve Volume* is the volume of air that can be inspired over and above the resting tidal volume. *Expiratory Reserve Volume* is the volume of air that can be forcibly expired after the resting tidal volume has been expired.

131. **The correct answer is (B).** *Surfactant* is secreted by Type II alveolar cells.

132. **The correct answer is (B).** In a mixture of gases, the pressure exerted by any one gas is known as *partial pressure* (Dalton's Law). The partial pressures of oxygen and carbon dioxide determine the direction that a gas moves through a respiratory membrane.

133. **The correct answer is (A).** Oxygen is weakly bound to hemoglobin to form oxyhemoglobin.

134. **The correct answer is (C).** Overall reaction: $CO_2 + H_2O \leftrightarrow H_2CO_3 \leftrightarrow H^+ + HCO_3^-$. Carbonic anhydrase present in erythrocytes catalyzes the rate-limiting first reaction.

135. **The correct answer is (B).** Erthropoietin is a hormonal substance that is formed especially in the kidney and stimulates red blood cell formation.

136. **The correct answer is (D).** *Micturition* is the process of expelling urine from the bladder.

137. **The correct answer is (B).** The kidney contains approximately 1 million functional units, nephrons.

138. **The correct answer is (B).** Hormonal control of sodium reabsorption occurs mainly in the collecting ducts.

139. **The correct answer is (B).** Human sex cells, sperm and egg, are haploid. Haploid cells contain half the full complement of chromosomes (i.e., 23 chromosomes).

140. **The correct answer is (D).** *Angiotensin* is involved in sodium reabsorption by the kidney.

141. **The correct answer is (C).** SNPs represent the most common form of genetic variant and are estimated to occur approximately every 1,000 base pairs.

142. The correct answer is (D). *Homozygotes* and *heterozygotes* may display the same phenotype. For example, in the case of the presence of a dominant allele, an individual carrying the dominant allele (either homozygote or heterozygote) will display the same phenotype.

143. The correct answer is (B). The higher the required activation energy, the lower the reaction rate.

144. The correct answer is (B). An enzyme affects the rate at which equilibrium is achieved. However, it cannot change the final equilibrium.

145. The correct answer is (C). Transfer RNA carries the appropriate amino acid to the ribosome during protein synthesis.

Quantitative Ability

146. The correct answer is (C). Multiplying numerators and denominators gives: $3 \times 6 = 18$ and $5 \times 8 = 40$, thus $\dfrac{3}{5} \times \dfrac{6}{8} = \dfrac{18}{40} = \dfrac{9}{20}$.

147. The correct answer is (A). Inverting and multiplying gives $\dfrac{2}{3} \times \dfrac{9}{4} = \dfrac{18}{12} = \dfrac{3}{2}$.

148. The correct answer is (B). A common denominator is $3 \times 8 = 24$. Then, $\dfrac{1}{3} = \dfrac{8}{24}, \dfrac{2}{8} = \dfrac{6}{24}$ and their sum is $\dfrac{14}{24} = \dfrac{7}{12}$.

149. The correct answer is (C). Using 30 as a common denominator gives: $\dfrac{24}{30} - \dfrac{12}{30} = \dfrac{12}{30} = \dfrac{2}{5}$.

150. The correct answer is (A). The product term is $\dfrac{1}{2} \times \dfrac{1}{2} = \dfrac{1}{4}$. Thus, $\dfrac{1}{4} + \dfrac{1}{4} = \dfrac{2}{4} = \dfrac{1}{2}$.

151. The correct answer is (D). Simple decimal number addition and subtraction.

152. The correct answer is (B). Decimal number multiplication and addition.

153. The correct answer is (A). Add the figures inside the parentheses and multiply by the 0.25 to get 2, then add 4 to get 6.

154. The correct answer is (D). Add the figures inside the parentheses and divide by 0.4 to get 30, then subtract 1 to get 29.

155. The correct answer is (B). The quotient of the terms in parentheses is $\dfrac{12}{6} = 2$, then multiply by 2.5 to get 5.

156. The correct answer is (B). Seventy-five percent is 75 out of 100, i.e., $75\% = \dfrac{75}{100} = 75\% = 0.75 = \dfrac{3}{4}$.

157. The correct answer is (C). The fraction $\frac{3}{5}$ corresponds to $\frac{60}{100} = 60\%$.

158. The correct answer is (A). 0.15×40 cookies = 6 cookies.

159. The correct answer is (D). Five to the third power = $5^3 = 5 \times 5 \times 5 = 125$. Then, $125 + 5 = 130$.

160. The correct answer is (A). For the two terms, $2 \times 2 \times 2 = 8$ and $2 \times 2 = 4$. Then, $8 \times 4 = 32$.

161. The correct answer is (B). When multiplying a number raised to an exponent (n) by the same number also raised to an exponent (m), add the exponents. Thus, $Y^n \times Y^m = Y^{(n+m)}$.

162. The correct answer is (D). In general, any number raised to a negative exponent is equal to the inverse of the number raised to the corresponding positive exponent, e.g., $Y^{-2} = \frac{1}{Y^2}$.

163. The correct answer is (D). Solve this problem by inspection. The cube root of 8 is 2, i.e., $2 \times 2 \times 2 = 8$.

164. The correct answer is (C). $\sqrt{2} \times \sqrt{6} \times \sqrt{3} = \sqrt{(2 \times 6 \times 3)} = \sqrt{36} = 6$

165. The correct answer is (B). The log of a number is the power to which the base of the log must be raised to obtain the number. Here, the base 5 must be raised to the second power to obtain 25.

166. The correct answer is (D). The factors of 55 are 5 and 11. The number 154 can be factored as 11×14, or $11 \times 7 \times 2$. The common factor of 55 and 154 is 11.

167. The correct answer is (D). A prime number is a whole number that cannot be divided by any other whole number but itself or 1.

168. The correct answer is (B). The square root of 49 is equal to 7, and thus not less than 7.

169. The correct answer is (A). The vertical bars instruct you to take the absolute (positive) value of the enclosed number. Thus, $13 - |-2| + |-6| = 13 - 2 + 6 = 17$.

170. The correct answer is (C). The expression illustrates different associations of the multipliers 5, 25, 8, and $(3 + 4)$.

171. The correct answer is (A). $5x + 13y - 6z = 5 \times 2 + 13 \times 3 - 6 \times 4 = 10 + 39 - 24 = 25$.

172. The correct answer is (D). $\dfrac{12 + \left[15 \times 2 - 7 \times 8 + 2\right]}{8} = \dfrac{12 + \left[-24\right]}{8} = 12 - 3 = 9$.

173. The correct answer is (B). $\dfrac{KL^2}{C} = 5 \times \dfrac{10^2}{2} = 5 \times \dfrac{100}{2} = 250$.

174. The correct answer is (B). The volume of a cylinder is obtained as the area of the circle that forms its base, πr^2, and its height, h. Cylinder volume = $\pi r^2 h$.

175. The correct answer is (D). Collecting terms in x on the left, $4x + 6x = 17 + 3$; $10x = 20$; $x = 2$.

176. The correct answer is (C). Multiply each side of the equation by the product of the denominators (lowest common denominator) to get $2(2y + 3) - 10 \times 10 = 5(4 - 3y)$, or $4y + 6 - 100 = 20 - 15y$. Collect terms in y on the left: $4y + 15y = 20 - 6 + 100$. Or, $19y = 114$, and thus $y = 6$.

177. The correct answer is (B). Multiplying to eliminate the parentheses: $z + 5 = 4z + 8 - 2z - 1$. Collect terms in z on the left: $z - 4z + 2z = 8 - 1 - 5$, or, $-z = 2$, $z = -2$.

178. The correct answer is (D). One has the two equations: $A = 4B$ and $A + B = 30$. Substituting the first into the second gives $4B + B = 30$, and thus $B = 6$. Using this in the first equation gives $A = 4 \times 6 = 24$.

179. The correct answer is (D). One has two equations: $J = 3H$ and $J - 4 = 5(H - 4)$. Substituting the first into the second gives $3H - 4 = 5H - 20$. Thus, $-2H = -16$, or $H = 8$. Substituting this into the first equation gives $J = 3 \times 8 = 24$.

180. The correct answer is (C). Let the initial speed be x mph. Then, $x \times 2\text{hrs.} + (x + 20) \times 4\text{hrs.} = 320$ miles. Thus, $2x + 4x + 80 = 320$. Or, $6x = 240$ and $x = 40$.

181. The correct answer is (A). Collecting terms in y on the left, $5y^2 - 10y = 0$. Factoring, $5y(y-2) = 0$. Therefore, $y = 0$ and $y = 2$.

182. The correct answer is (A). Collecting terms in Z on the left gives: $aZ - cZ = d + b$, or, $Z(a - c) = d + b$, and $Z = \dfrac{d+b}{a-c}$.

183. The correct answer is (D). Collecting terms in A on the left: $8A - 3A > -7 + 17$, or, $5A > 10$, and $A > 2$.

184. The correct answer is (B). Multiply all terms by $6 \times 4 = 24$ to clear the denominators: $4B - 6B \geq 24$, so $-2B \geq 24$ and $-B \geq 12$. Multiply by -1 and reverse the inequality to get $B \leq -12$.

185. The correct answer is (C). Collect terms in C on the left: $3C - 8C < -3 + 18$, or $-5C < 15$ and $-C < 3$. Multiply by -1 and reverse the equality to get: $C > -3$.

186. The correct answer is (B). The equation can be factored to give $(y + 5)(y + 2) = 0$. Each factor can be equated to zero, thus, $y + 5 = 0$ and $y + 2 = 0$. Accordingly, the solutions are $y = -5$ and $y = -2$.

187. The correct answer is (C). The equation is factored. Each term can be set equal to zero. Thus, $x = 0$ and $x - 12 = 0$. The solutions are $x = 0$ and $x = 12$.

188. The correct answer is (A). Collecting all terms on the left: $K^2 - 5K^2 + 36 = 0$ or, $4K^2 - 36 = 0$ and $K^2 = 9$. Thus, $K = 3$ and $K = -3$.

189. The correct answer is (D). Adding the equations gives: $0B + 6C = 12$. Thus, $C = 2$.

190. The correct answer is (A). Multiply the second equation by 2 and subtract it from the first to get: $3B = -9$ or $B = -3$.

191. The correct answer is (B). Multiply the first equation by 2 and add to the second to get: $11R + 0S = 44$ or, $R = 4$.

192. The correct answer is (D). The patient will take 3 tablets each day. Thus, x tablets is to 14 days as 3 tablets is to 1 day, i.e., $\dfrac{x}{14} = \dfrac{3}{1}$ and $x = 3 \times \dfrac{14}{1} = 42$.

193. The correct answer is (C). Let x grams be the amount required to make 50 milliliters.

Then, $\dfrac{x \text{ grams}}{50 \text{ milliliters}} = \dfrac{16 \text{ grams}}{200 \text{ milliliters}}$.

Accordingly, $x = \dfrac{(50 \text{ml}. \times 16 \text{g}.)}{200 \text{ml}.} = 4\text{g}$.

194. The correct answer is (A). A 10 percent mixture will contain 10 grams of coal tar per 100 grams of the mixture. Let x grams be the amount of coal tar to be mixed with 450 grams of zinc oxide paste. The total weight of the mixture will be $(450 + x)$ grams. Accordingly, $\dfrac{10 \text{ grams}}{100 \text{ grams}} = \dfrac{x \text{ grams}}{(450+x)}$.

Solve this equation for x: $10 \times (450 + x) = 100x$; $4,500 = 100x - 10x = 90x$; $x = \dfrac{4,500}{90} = 50$.

195. The correct answer is (C). The average, or arithmetic mean, of a set of N numbers is obtained by summing the numbers and dividing by N. In this problem, the sum is 410 and N = 5. Thus, the average is 82.

196. The correct answer is (B). The median of a set of numbers is the number in the middle when the numbers are arranged in order. Here, the ordered numbers are: 62, 72, 77, 86, 93, 96, and 98. The middle number—the fourth number—is 86.

197. The correct answer is (A). A triangle with two sides equal is an isosceles triangle with angles A and B equal. The sum of the three angles must equal 180°, i.e., 180° = A + B + 30° = 2A + 30°.

Or, $A = \dfrac{(180° - 30°)}{2} = \dfrac{150°}{2} = 75°$.

198. The correct answer is (C). The diagonal of a rectangle together with the sides forms a right triangle. For a right triangle, the sum of the squares of the two sides forming the right angle is equal to the square of the opposite side (here, the diagonal). Thus, $d^2 = (6\text{cm}.)^2 + (8\text{cm}.)^2 = 100\text{cm}.^2$. Thus, $d = \sqrt{(100\text{cm}.^2} = 10\text{cm}$.

199. The correct answer is (B). The diameter of the circle is equal to the length of the sides of the square, 8 inches. The area, A, of a circle is given by $A = \pi r^2 = \pi\left[\dfrac{d}{2}\right]^2 = \pi\dfrac{d^2}{4} = 3.14 \times \dfrac{64}{4} = 50.2$ square inches.

200. The correct answer is (D). Note that $\beta + 45 = 180$. Because lines A and B are parallel, $\alpha = \beta$, and thus $a + 45° = 180°$. Accordingly, $\alpha = 180° - 45° = 135°$.

201. The correct answer is (D). In this problem, there are two unknowns and sufficient information is provided to set up two equations: $B = 4A$ and Area $= 100 = A \times B$. Substituting the first into the second gives: $100 = A \times 4A = 4A^2$. Then, $A = \left(\dfrac{100}{4}\right)^{\frac{1}{2}} = 5$. Thus, $B = 4$ and $A = 20$.

202. The correct answer is (B). The diagonal of the square is equal to the diameter of the circle (10). Using the Pythagorean Theorem, we can obtain the length of the sides (A) of the square: $(10)^2 = A^2 + A^2 = 2A^2$, or, $A^2 = 50$. But, the area of the square is $A \times A = A^2$.

203. The correct answer is (A). The distance between two points can be obtained using the formula (derived from the Pythagorean Theorem): $d = \left[\left(x1 - x2\right)^2 + \left(y1 - y2\right)^2\right]^{\frac{1}{2}}$. Here, $d = \left[\left(-3-1\right)^2 + \left(2+1\right)^2\right]^{\frac{1}{2}} = \left[16+9\right]^{\frac{1}{2}} = 5$.

204. The correct answer is (D). The perimeter is given by the sum of the sides: $270 = AB + AC + BC = 35 + 150 + BC$. Thus, $BC = 270 - 185 = 85$.

205. The correct answer is (C). The volume of a cube will be equal to the length of a side cubed. Since the volume is 1,000, the length of each side is 10. The area of a single face is $10 \times 10 = 100$. There are six faces, thus the surface area is $6 \times 100 = 600$.

206. The correct answer is (C). The x-intercept is the value of x when $y = 0$. Thus, $0 = 5x + 25$ or, $x = \dfrac{-25}{5} = -5$.

207. The correct answer is (A). The equation for a straight line can be obtained using the coordinates for any two points on the line. Here, we may note that at $X = 20$, $Y = 75$ and at $X = 40$, $Y = 125$. Since the slope of a straight line is constant, one can utilize the relationship: $\dfrac{(Y-Y_1)}{(X-X_1)} = \dfrac{(Y_2-Y_1)}{(X_2-X_1)}$. Putting in the values for the two point's gives: $\dfrac{Y-75}{X-20} = \dfrac{125-75}{40-20} = \dfrac{50}{20}$.

Solving for Y gives $Y-75 = (X-20) \times \dfrac{50}{20}$. Or, $20Y - 1{,}500 = 50X - 1{,}000$; therefore, $Y = 2.5X + 25$.

208. The correct answer is (C). The slope of a straight line is calculated as the ratio of a segment length along the ordinate ($y_2 - y_1$) to the corresponding segment length along the abscissa ($x_2 - x_1$). Thus, if we take the ordinate segment to be from 50 to 150, the corresponding abscissa segment is from 1 to 3 and the ratio of their lengths is $\dfrac{150-50}{3-1} = \dfrac{100}{2} = 50$. Thus, the slope is 50, indicating a driving speed of 50 miles per hour.

209. The correct answer is (C). Twenty-five percent, or one-fourth, of the town's pets are dogs. Since there are 5,000 dogs, there are 20,000 pets total. Birds represent 15 percent of the total and, therefore, number in total 3,000.

210. The correct answer is (C). The vertical bar at 2000 indicates that $650 million was spent in that year, while the vertical bar at 2002 indicates $400 million was spent. The difference is $250 million.

Chemistry

211. The correct answer is (C). nM is a short notation for nanomolarity, and it equals to 10^{-9} M. 10^{-3} M equals to 1 mM, 10^{-6} M equals to 1 μM and 10^{-12} M equals to 1 pM.

212. The correct answer is (D). The mole molecular weight of NaOH is 40; therefore, 1 mol. of NaOH weighs 40 grams. The solution contains $0.5L \times \dfrac{0.3\text{mol.}}{L} = 0.15\text{mol.}$ NaOH, and the amount of NaOH needed is $0.15\text{mol.} \times \dfrac{40\text{g.}}{\text{mol.}} = 6$ grams.

213. The correct answer is (B). Total amount of NaCl in the final solution equals to $0.5L \times \dfrac{1\text{mol.}}{L} + 0.2L \times \dfrac{2\text{mol.}}{L} = 0.9\text{mol.}$; therefore the final concentration will be $\dfrac{0.9\text{mol.}}{2L} = 0.45M$.

214. The correct answer is (C). An acidic solution has pH < 7, while a basic solution has pH > 7. When pH = 7, the solution is neutral.

215. **The correct answer is (A).** For an addition or a subtraction, the result should have the same precision as the *least* precise measurement. The number with greatest uncertainty is 10.3, therefore, the answer should be rounded to the nearest tenth, 14.8. For multiplication or division, the answer must contain the same number of significant figures as in the measurement that has the least number of significant figures.

216. **The correct answer is (D).** For a neutral atom, the number of electrons must equal to the number of protons. The number of neutrons only affects the mass of the atom, but does not have direct relationship to the number of electrons.

217. **The correct answer is (C).** Isotopes only differ in their mass—they have the same number of protons and electrons. The isotopes of an element have the same chemical properties and this is the base for isotope labeling widely used in chemistry and biological researches.

218. **The correct answer is (A).** The hydrocarbon containing seven carbon atoms is called heptane. Pentane contains 5 carbons, octane contains 8 carbons, and decane contains 10 carbons.

219. **The correct answer is (C).** The two carbons in ethylene are connected by a double bond that cannot freely rotate. The carbon has sp^2 hybrid orbitals, which is planar in geometry.

220. **The correct answer is (A).** Methlyene group is CH_2 and methine group is CH. Methane is the simplest hydrocarbon molecule.

221. **The correct answer is (D).** R from the Latin *rectus* meaning right and S from the Latin *sinister*, meaning left. R and S are used to assign the absolute configuration of chiral centers in a molecule.

222. **The correct answer is (C).** Both oxygen and nitrogen have sp^3 hybrid orbitals. Oxygen in water molecule has two lone pairs to occupy the remaining two oribitals. Nitrogen atom in ammonia has one lone pair.

223. **The correct answer is (B).** There are two hydrogen atoms in H_2O_2. The molecular weight of H_2O_2 is 34, therefore, the percent composition by mass for hydrogen is $\frac{2}{34} = 0.059 = 5.9\%$.

224. **The correct answer is (A).** Chlorous acid is $HClO_2$, chloric acid is $HClO_3$, and perchloric acid is $HClO_4$.

225. **The correct answer is (D).** A chemical equation must obey the law of conservation of matter. The number of atoms in reactants must equal the number of atoms in the product. The number of oxygen atoms is not balance in choices (A) and (B). The numbers of K and Cl are not balanced in choice (C). Only in choice (D) are all the atoms balanced properly.

226. **The correct answer is (B).** Strong acids, strong bases, and ionic salts are all strong electrolytes. Weak acids and weak bases are normally weak electrolytes. Acetic acid is a weak acid.

227. **The correct answer is (C).** Brønsted acid is a proton donor and Brønsted base is a proton acceptor. $H_2PO_4^-$ can accept a proton to become H_3PO_4 or release a proton to become HPO_4^{2-}. Therefore, it can act as either an acid or a base.

228. The correct answer is (B). Ca gives up electrons to oxygen in the reaction; therefore it is a reducing agent. Oxygen gains electrons in the reaction, and its oxidation number changed from 0 to -2. The product is solid CaO, which has much lower entropy than the gaseous oxygen.

229. The correct answer is (A). One atm and 0°C is the standard condition, at which 1 mole of gas occupies 22.4 liters of volume. One gram of hydrogen gas is 0.5mol., therefore the volume it occupies at standard condition is 11.2 liters.

230. The correct answer is (A). It tests the understanding Graham's law of effusion: The rates of effusion of two gases at the same temperature and pressure are inversely proportional to the square roots of their densities or molar masses. Oxygen has a larger molar mass than nitrogen; therefore nitrogen has a higher effusion rate.

231. The correct answer is (D). For principle quantum number n, the maximum number of electrons can be present is $2n^2$. For $n = 2$, this is 8.

232. The correct answer is (B). Pauli exclusion principle.

233. The correct answer is (C). The nitrogen atoms in NH_3 has sp^3 hybrid orbital, thus NH_3 is tetrahedral in geometry with a lone pair occupies one corner. All other molecules in the choice have planar geometry.

234. The correct answer is (A). Choices (B) and (C) have a carbonyl group that contains a pi bond. Naphthalene is a fused-ring aromatic hydrocarbon that contains a pi bond. Only CH_3OH does not contain any pi bond.

235. The correct answer is (D). A hydrogen bond is a chemical bond that is formed between polar molecules that contain hydrogen covalently bonded to a small, highly electronegative atom such as fluorine, oxygen or nitrogen. Carbon usually cannot form hydrogen bond due to its low electronegative property.

236. The correct answer is (D). Two acetic acid molecules can form a dimer via hydrogen bonding. This dimer is much less polar compared with a single acetic acid molecule, hence it is soluble to nonpolar solvents. It is not an aromatic compound, nor it can react with benzene under normal conditions.

237. The correct answer is (C). The *homolysis* process is based on osmosis, in which water diffuses from a dilute solution or water through a semipermeable membrane into a solution of higher concentration. Since water moves into the cell, the solution is more dilute than that inside the cell; therefore it is a *hypotonic* solution. A *hypertonic* solution has a higher concentration while an isotonic solution has equal concentration compared with that of the other side of the semipermeable membrane.

238. The correct answer is (D). K_w is essentially an equilibrium constant, therefore it is dependent on temperature. It does not depend pH (which indicates the concentration of proton) of the solution. It does not depend on pressure since the system is in solution state.

239. The correct answer is (B). At 25°C, pH + pOH = pK_w = 14, hence pOH =10, and [OH⁻] = 10^{-10}M.

240. The correct answer is (A). The *stronger* the acid is, the *weaker* its conjugate base.

241. The correct answer is (D). For oxioacids that have the same central atom but different numbers of attached groups, the acid strength increases as the oxidation number of the central atom increases. The oxidation numbers are +1, choice (A), +3, choice (B), +5, choice (C), and +7, choice (D).

242. The correct answer is (C). CaO forms base $Ca(OH)_2$ with water. All others form acids when react with water.

243. The correct answer is (B). The maximum possible concentration of [H⁺] in a 0.1M solution of HA is 0.1M. For strong acid, this is true. For weak acid, the [H⁺] is much less than 0.1M due to incomplete dissociation. Therefore the pH is larger than 1.

244. The correct answer is (A). The solution is basic. This salt is formed by a weak acid HCN with a weak base NH_3. Both of the anion (CN⁻) and cation (NH4⁺) will undergo hydrolysis in water. Since K_b >> Ka, the anion hydrolysis that produces [OH⁻] will be more extensive than the cation hydrolysis that produces [H_3O^+].

245. The correct answer is (B). A buffer solution is a solution of a weak acid or base and its salt. $HClO_4$ is a very strong acid—hence this acid and its salt can not make a buffer system.

246. The correct answer is (D). When water vapor becomes water, the water molecules are more ordered. Since entropy is a direct measure of the randomness or disorder of a system, for the same molar amount of substance, it is always true that $S_{solid} < S_{liquid} << S_{gas}$.

247. The correct answer is (B). Mercury has both +1 (mercurous) and +2 (mercuric) oxidation numbers in its compounds.

248. The correct answer is (D). Fluorine is an exception since it is the most electronegative element. It can only have two oxidation numbers, 0 (as in F_2) and –1, in its compounds.

249. The correct answer is (A). Hydrogen peroxide is not a planar molecule. Since it can form hydrogen bonding with water, it is miscible with water easily. The oxidation number is –1 in hydrogen peroxide, in the middle of –2 (such as in MgO) and 0 (in O_2), hence it can act as either oxidation or reducing agent.

250. The correct answer is (C). The atomic mass does not change, so only an electron is emitted.

251. The correct answer is (D). Atoms in triple bonds are fixed with the pi bonds and are not allowed to freely rotate.

252. The correct answer is (B). The three structural isomers are: $CH_3CH_2CH_2CH_2CH_3$, $CH_3CH_2CH(CH_3)_2$, and $C(CH_3)_4$.

253. The correct answer is (C). *R-* and *S-* are used to assign absolute configuration in chiral atoms in a molecule. *Ortho-* and *para-* are used for positions in aromatic rings, and *n-*and *t-* is used for hydrocarbon branching.

254. The correct answer is (D). It does not have the general ester functional group of RCOOR'.

255. The correct answer is (A). H_2S is hydrogen sulfide. Choices (C) and (D) do not exist.

256. The correct answer is (B). Avogadro's law and Boyle's law has nothing to do with chemical reaction mechanisms, while Saytzeff's rule deals with dehydration.

257. The correct answer is (A). The oxidation state of carbon is 4 in CO_2, -2 in CH_3OH, 2 in HCOOH, and 0 in CH_4, respectively.

258. The correct answer is (B). The -OH group from the carboxylic acid and the -H in hydroxyl group of the alcohol form water molecule in the esterification reaction.

259. The correct answer is (D). Phenol is a stronger acid than methanol due to the stabilization effect from the aromatic ring when it losses a proton. However, it is not as acidic as acetic acid.

260. The correct answer is (D). Tollens' test for aldehydes is based on the ability of silver ions to oxidize aldehydes. Ketones, esters, and amines cannot be oxidized under this condition.

261. The correct answer is (C). The maximum number of possible stereoisomers is 2^n, where n is the number of non-identical asymmetric carbon atoms.

262. The correct answer is (B). Sucrose is sweeter than glucose. Glucose contains asymmetric carbons and it is optically active. It contains aldehyde group; hence it gives positive Tollens' test and can be reduced to alcohol by hydrogen.

263. The correct answer is (A). Amino acids have the general formula of $RCHNH_2COOH$. They can be classified as neutral amino acids when their molecules have the same number of amino and carboxyl groups, as acids when their molecules have more carboxyl groups than amino groups, or as basic when their molecules have more amino groups than carboxyl groups. In the choices given, only glycine has the same number of carboxyl and amino group. Lysine, arginine and histidine all have more extra amino groups and are classified as basic amino acids.

264. The correct answer is (C). Amides have the general formula of $R-CO-NH_2$, and the $-NH_2$ can be $-NHR$ or $-NR_2$. $R-CO-NR_3$ has an extra R group attached to the nitrogen.

265. The correct answer is (B). Trichlorbenzene can have three isomers, 1, 2, 3-; 1, 2, 4-; and 1, 3, 5-trichlorbenzene. Another arrangement is essentially equivalent to one of these three isomers.

266. **The correct answer is (D).** Diels–Alder reaction is the addition of an alkene (which is called the dienophile) to a diene to form a cyclohexene. It is the most important cycloaddition reaction from the point of view of synthesis. A carboxylic acid and an alcohol can react to form an ester; an alkene and a halogen can have addition reaction; an acid and a base is a acid–base neutralization reaction.

267. **The correct answer is (A).** Esters have the general formula of R–CO–OR'. ROR' are ethers, RCOR' are ketones and ROH are alcohols.

268. **The correct answer is (C).** Fatty acids and steroids belong to *lipids*. Cholesterols belong to *steroids*. Starch, however, belong to *carbohydrates*, not lipids.

269. **The correct answer is (A).** A primary amine has the general formula of RNH_2. A secondary amine has the general formula of R_2NH and a tertiary amine has the general formula of R_3N.

270. **The correct answer is (B).** The α-helix and β-sheet are two examples of protein secondary structure. The primary structure of a protein refers to the number, kind, and sequences of amino acid units composing the polypeptide chain or chains. The secondary structure refers to the regular, three-dimensional structure held together by hydrogen bonding between the carbonyl oxygen and the amino hydrogen in the polypeptide chains. The tertiary structure normally refers to the overall shape of a protein.

PART V

Pharmacy Licensure

Chapter 12: Licensure Requirements

INTERN LICENSE

Upon registration in a pharmacy college/school, students are eligible to become pharmacy interns. Since some states require that interns be licensed, check with the Dean's office of your college/school concerning internship requirements in your state. All states require a minimum of 1,500 internship hours under the guidance of a pharmacy preceptor licensed in the state in which the student is registered. These hours may be obtained during summer breaks between professional years in the college of pharmacy, breaks during the academic year, or after graduation. While some state boards of pharmacy require that a minimum number of these hours be obtained after graduation, the current trend is to complete the hours beforehand so that you can take the state board of pharmacy examination to become licensed upon graduation.

A number of boards of pharmacy give students credit for the entire 1,500 hours of internship during the clinical curriculum of a college/school of pharmacy. Some boards of pharmacy only give 400 hours, while other boards recognize the clinical experience in the Pharm.D. program for the entire internship-hour requirements. For information on how many hours of internship will be granted, and on the specific areas of practice allowed for internship credit, contact your state board. A listing of state boards of pharmacy follows later in this chapter.

PHARMACY LICENSE REQUIREMENTS

After graduation, you must take a theoretical and practical examination administered by a state board of pharmacy. The National Association of Boards of Pharmacy's standardized North American Pharmacist Licensure Examination (NABPLEX) is administered by all state boards of pharmacy, with the exception of California. (California conducts its own licensure examination.)The NABPLEX is administered several times a year; each state board adheres to a standardized set of dates for giving the exam. These dates can be obtained from each state board of pharmacy office.

NABPLEX Examination

One of the most important functions of boards of pharmacy is to protect the public health and welfare. Each state board must set standards of competence for the practice of pharmacy. State laws require the assessment of the proficiency of each candidate in the knowledge, skills, and abilities necessary for the practice of pharmacy. State boards use the NABPLEX to make that assessment. A candidate for licensure who passes this examination is judged to have the required proficiency in that state and can also practice pharmacy in other licensing jurisdictions that offer reciprocity.

The licensing examination, which is oriented toward professional practice, is a qualifying evaluation rather than a competitive test. The NABPLEX Review Committee established standards of knowledge, skills, and abilities they consider essential for the practice of pharmacy. NABPLEX is used to assess these standards and is one determinant of a candidate's qualification for licensure. By nature, the examination emphasizes that facts and information are meaningless without the ability to apply them in a practical situation. Furthermore, it highlights skills and abilities that must be maintained throughout the candidate's professional career.

The NAPLEX is a computer-adaptive test used by the state boards of pharmacy as part of their assessment of a candidate's competence to practice pharmacy. It consists of 185 multiple-choice test questions. (150 questions are used to calculate your test score while the other thirty-five items are pretest questions that do not affect your NAPLEX score.) The questions cover all aspects of pharmacy, with a majority of the questions asked in a scenario-based format (i.e., patient profiles with accompanying test questions). The exam is administered three times per year in January, June, and October, at specific computer centers across the country.

RECIPROCITY BETWEEN STATES

Reciprocity is the process of transferring a license from one state to another. Most states recognize test scores from other states with some exceptions, such as California, which requires pharmacists to take its own board of pharmacy examination before becoming licensed. Typically, upon completing the state board of pharmacy requirements of a particular state, you must practice one year before being able to reciprocate your license in another state. While each state law is different, many states participate in the score transfer program, which transfers the NABPLEX test scores to another state.

In order to reciprocate to another state, you must fill out the appropriate forms from the National Association of Boards of Pharmacy and from the individual state board offices. Most state boards of pharmacy also require a law examination along with the reciprocation papers. (The examination is on the federal and state laws governing pharmacy practice.) Specific information on reciprocation among various states can be obtained from the National Association of Boards of Pharmacy, 700 Busse Highway, Park Ridge, IL 60068; phone: (847) 698-6227 or fax: (847) 698-0124; e-mail: ceo@nabp.net and/or the individual state board of pharmacy. See the Appendix for contact information for each state pharmacy board.

RE-LICENSURE REQUIREMENTS

Requirements for re-licensure vary by state. However, most states require mandatory continuing education. As of January 2003, fifty-two of the fifty-three boards of pharmacy require continuing education for re-licensure, with the exception of Hawaii. See the list on the following page for the boards that require continuing education.

State Boards That Require Continuing Education

Alabama	Louisiana	Oklahoma
Alaska	Maine	Oregon
Arizona	Maryland	Pennsylvania
Arkansas	Massachusetts	Puerto Rico
California	Michigan	Rhode Island
Colorado	Minnesota	South Carolina
Connecticut	Mississippi	South Dakota
Delaware	Missouri	Tennessee
District of Columbia	Montana	Texas
Florida	Nebraska	Utah
Georgia	Nevada	Vermont
Guam	New Hampshire	Virginia
Idaho	New Jersey	Washington
Illinois	New Mexico	West Virginia
Indiana	New York	Wisconsin
Iowa	North Carolina	Wyoming
Kansas	North Dakota	
Kentucky	Ohio	

The number of hours of continuing education required range from a minimum of 10-contact hours per year to 30-contact hours every two years. Continuing education credits are defined in the following manner: One continuing education unit (1.0 CEU) equals 10-contact hours of credit. Pharmacists are required to report the continuing education programs they attend to their boards of pharmacy.

The ACPE evaluates and approves providers of pharmacy continuing education through a provider approval program. The purpose of this program is to assure pharmacists of the quality of continuing education programs. The provider approval program is also designed to do the following:

1. Advance the quality of continuing education, thereby advancing the practice of pharmacy.

2. Establish criteria and characteristics of approved continuing pharmaceutical education programs.

3. Provide pharmacists with a dependable basis for selecting continuing education programs.

4. Provide a basis for uniform acceptance of continuing education credits among the states.

5. Provide feedback to providers about their offerings, encouraging periodic self-evaluation with a view toward continual improvement and strengthening of continuing education activities. A pamphlet describing the standards for assessing and approving continuing education programs, as well as a list of approved continuing education programs, can be obtained from the American Council on Pharmaceutical Education (ACPE), One East Wacker Drive, Chicago, IL 60601.

APPENDIX

DIRECTORY OF ACCREDITED COLLEGES AND SCHOOLS OF PHARMACY

This is a list of accredited schools as of this printing. Note that there are schools pending accreditation; check with the college/school you are applying to in order to verify status if they do not appear on this list.

Alabama

Auburn University
Office of Academic & Student Affairs
Harrison School of Pharmacy
209 Pharmacy Building
Auburn, AL 36849-5501
Phone: (334) 844-8348
Fax: (334) 844-8353
Web site: pharmacy.auburn.edu
(PCAT REQUIRED)

Samford University
McWhorter School of Pharmacy
800 Lakeshore Drive
Birmingham, AL 35229-7027
Phone: (205) 726-2820
Fax: (205) 726-3759
Web site: www.samford.edu/schools/pharmacy.html

Arizona

University of Arizona
College of Pharmacy
P.O. Box 210207
Tucson, AZ 85721-0207
Phone: (520) 626-1427
Fax: (520) 626-4063
Web site: www.pharmacy.arizona.edu/news/
011801.shtml
(PCAT REQUIRED)

Midwestern University
College of Pharmacy
The Office of Admissions
19555 North 59th Avenue
Glendale, AZ 85308
Phone: (800) 458-6253 or (602) 572-3215
E-mail: admiss@midwestern.edu
Web site: www.midwestern.edu/ccp/
(PCAT REQUIRED)

Arkansas

University of Arkansas Medical Sciences Campus
College of Pharmacy
4301 West Markham Street—Slot 522
Little Rock, AR 72205-7122
Phone: (501) 686-5557
Fax: (501) 686-8315
Web site: www.uams.edu/cop

California

University of California
School of Pharmacy
Student Affairs, Box 0150
San Francisco, CA 94143-0150
Phone: (415) 476-1225
Fax: (415) 476-0688
Web site: pharmacy.ucsf.edu/

University of the Pacific
Thomas J. Long School of Pharmacy and Health Sciences
3601 Pacific Avenue
Stockton, CA 95211
Phone: (209) 946-2561
Fax: (209) 946-2410
Web site: www.uop.edu/pharmacy/index.html

University of Southern California
School of Pharmacy
Office of Admissions and Student Affairs
1985 Zonal Avenue
Los Angeles, CA 90033-1086
Phone: (213) 342-1369
Fax: (213) 342-1681
Web site: www.usc.edu/hsc/pharmacy/index.html

Western University of Health Sciences College of Pharmacy
College Plaza
309 East Second Street
Pomona, CA 91766-1889
Phone: (909) 469-5369
Fax: (909) 469-5501
Web site: www.westernu.edu

Colorado

University of Colorado
School of Pharmacy/C238
4299 East Ninth Ave.
Denver, CO 80262-0238
Phone: (303) 270-5055
Fax: (303) 270-6281
Web site: www.uchsc.edu/sop/

Connecticut

School of Pharmacy
University of Connecticut
BOX U-92/372 Fairfield Road
Storrs, CT 06269-2092
Phone: (860) 486-2115
Fax: (860) 486-4998
E-mail: gerald@uconnvm.uconn.edu
Web site: www.ucc.uconn.edu/~wwwpharm/

District of Columbia

Howard University
College of Pharmacy, Nursing, and AHS
2300 4th Street NW
Washington, D.C. 20059
Phone: (202) 806-6452/6453
Fax: (202) 806-4636
Web site: www.howard.edu/HU-HomePages/schools/
pharm.html
(PCAT REQUIRED)

Florida

Florida A&M University
College of Pharmacy and Pharmaceutical Sciences
201 Dyson Pharmacy Building
Tallahassee, FL 32307-3800
Phone: (904) 599-3593
Fax: (904) 599-3447
Web site: www.famu.edu/acad/colleges/copps

Nova Southeastern University
College of Pharmacy
Health Professions Division
3200 South University Drive
Fort Lauderdale, FL 33328
Phone: (954) 262-1300
Fax: (954) 262-2278
Web site: www.nova.edu/cwis/centers/hpd/pharmacy
(PCAT REQUIRED)

College of Pharmacy
University of Florida
Box 100484
J. Hillis Miller Health Science Center
Gainesville, FL 32610-0484
Phone: (352) 392-9713
Fax: (352) 392-3480
Web site: www.cop.uf.edu/
(PCAT REQUIRED)

College of Pharmacy
Palm Beach Atlantic University
P.O. Box 24708
West Palm Beach, FL 33416
Phone: (561) 803-2000
Fax: (561) 803-2703
Web site: cosmas.pbac.edu/pharmacy

Georgia

College of Pharmacy
The University of Georgia
D. W. Brooks Drive
Athens, GA 30602-2351
Phone: (706) 542-1911
Fax: (706) 542-5269
Web site: www.rx.uga.edu
(PCAT REQUIRED)

Mercer University
Southern School of Pharmacy
3001 Mercer University Drive
Atlanta, GA 30341-4155
Phone: (770) 986-3300
Fax: (770) 986-3315
E-mail: matthews_h@atl1.mercer.edu
Web site: www.mercer.edu/pharmacy/
(PCAT REQUIRED)

Idaho

Idaho State University
College of Pharmacy
Campus Box 8288
970 South 5th Street
Pocatello, ID 83209-8288
Phone: (208) 282-4597
Fax: (208) 236-4482
Web site: www.pharmacy.isu.edu
(PCAT REQUIRED)

Illinois

Chicago College of Pharmacy
Midwestern University
555 31st Street
Downers Grove, IL 60515-1235
Phone: (800) 458-6258 or (630) 971-6417
Fax: (630) 971-6097
Web site: www.midwestern.edu/ccp/
(PCAT REQUIRED)

University of Illinois at Chicago
College of Pharmacy (M/C 874)
833 South Wood Street
Chicago, IL 60612-7230
Phone: (312) 996-7240
Fax: (312) 996-3273
Web site: www.uic.edu/pharmacy
(PCAT REQUIRED)

Indiana

Butler University
College of Pharmacy & Health Sciences
4600 Sunset Avenue
Indianapolis, IN 46208
Phone: (800) 368-6852
Fax: (317) 940-9930
E-mail: info@butler.edu
Web site: www.butler.edu
(PCAT REQUIRED)

Purdue University
School of Pharmacy and Pharmacal Sciences
1330 Heine Pharmacy Building
West Lafayette, IN 47907-1330
Phone: (765) 494-1368
Fax: (765) 494-7880
E-mail: chipr@pharmacy.purdue.edu
Web site: www.pharmacy.purdue.edu

Iowa

Drake University
College of Pharmacy & Health Sciences
2507 and University Avenue
Des Moines, IA 50311-4505
Phone: (800) 44-DRAKE or (515) 271-2172
Fax: (515) 271-4171
(PCAT REQUIRED)

University of Iowa
College of Pharmacy
115 South Grand Avenue
Iowa City, IA 52242
Phone: (319) 335-8794
Fax: (319) 353-5594
Web site: www.uiowa.edu/pharmacy/
(PCAT REQUIRED)

Kansas

University of Kansas
School of Pharmacy
2056 Malott Hall
Lawrence, KS 66045-2500
Phone: (785) 864-3591
Fax: (785) 864-5265
E-mail: jfincham@ukans.edu
Web site: www.pharm.ku.edu/dean
(PCAT REQUIRED)

Kentucky

University of Kentucky
College of Pharmacy
907 Rose Street
101 Pharmacy Building
Lexington, KY 40536-0082
Phone: (859) 323-6163
Fax: (859) 257-2128
Web site: www.mc.uky.edu/pharmacy
(PCAT REQUIRED)

Louisiana

Northeast Louisiana University
School of Pharmacy
700 University Avenue, Sugar Hall
Monroe, LA 71209-0470
Phone: (318) 342-1600
Fax: (318) 342-1606
E-mail: pybourn@alpha.ulm.edu
Web site: rxweb.ulm.edu/pharmacy/

Xavier University of Louisiana
College of Pharmacy
7325 Palmetto Street
New Orleans, LA 70125
Phone: (504) 483-7424
Fax: (504) 485-7930
Web site: www.xula.edu/pharmacy.html

Maryland

University of Maryland
School of Pharmacy
20 North Pine Street
Baltimore, MD 21201-1180
Phone: (410) 706-7650
Fax: (410) 706-4012
Web site: www.pharmacy.umaryland.edu/
(PCAT REQUIRED)

Massachusetts

Massachusetts College of Pharmacy and Health Sciences
179 Longwood Avenue
Boston, MA 02115-5896
Phone: (617) 732-2800 or outside MA (800) 225-5506
Fax: (617) 732-2244
Web site: www.mcp.edu/

Massachusetts College of Pharmacy and Health Sciences-
Worcester
19 Foster Street
Worcester, MA 01608
Phone: (508) 890-8855
Web site: www.mcp.edu/

Bouve College of Health Sciences
Northeastern University
School of Pharmacy
360 Huntington Avenue
206 Mugar Life Science Building
Boston, MA 02115
Phone: (617) 373-3380
Fax: (617) 373-7655
Web site: www.neu.edu/bouve/pharmacy

Michigan

Ferris State University
College of Pharmacy
220 Ferris Drive
Big Rapids, MI 49307-2740
Phone: (231) 591-3780
Fax: (231) 591-3829
Web site: www.ferris.edu/htmls/colleges/pharmacy/
(PCAT REQUIRED)

University of Michigan
College of Pharmacy
428 Church Street
Ann Arbor, MI 48109-1065
Phone: (734) 764-7312
Fax: (734) 763-2022
Web site: www.umich.edu/~pharmacy/

Wayne State University
College of Pharmacy and Allied Health Professions
105 Shapero Hall
Detroit, MI 48202-3489
Phone: (313) 577-1574
Fax: (313) 577-5589
Web site: wizard.pharm.wayne.edu
(PCAT REQUIRED)

Minnesota

University of Minnesota
College of Pharmacy
5-130 Weaver-Densford Hall
308 Harvard Street SE
Minneapolis, MN 55455-0343
Phone: (612) 624-1900
Fax: (612) 624-2974
E-mail: mspeedie@mailbox.mail.umn.edu
Web site: www.pharmacy.umn.edu

Mississippi

University of Mississippi
School of Pharmacy
Faser Hall
University, MS 38677-9814
Phone: (662) 915-7265
Fax: (662) 915-5704
Web site: www.olemiss.edu/depts/clph
(PCAT REQUIRED)

Missouri

St. Louis College of Pharmacy
4588 Parkview Place
St. Louis, MO 63110-1088
Phone: (314) 367-8700, Ext. 1072
Fax: (314) 367-2784
Web site: www.sticop.edu
(PCAT RECOMMENDED)

University of Missouri–Kansas City
School of Pharmacy
Katz Pharmacy Building
5005 Rockhill Road
Kansas City, MO 64110-2499
Phone: (816) 235-1607
Fax: (816) 235-5190
Web site: www.umkc.edu/pharmacy
(PCAT REQUIRED)

Montana

University of Montana
School of Pharmacy and Allied Health Sciences
32 Campus Drive #1512
Missoula, MT 59812-1512
Phone: (406) 243-4621
Fax: (406) 243-4209
E-mail: pharmacy@selway.umt.edu
Web site: www.umt.edu/pharmacy/
(PCAT REQUIRED)

Nebraska

Creighton University
School of Pharmacy & Health Professions
2500 California Street
Omaha, NE 68178-0401
Phone: (800) 325-2830 or (402) 280-2950
Fax: (402) 280-5738
Web site: spahp.creighton.edu/

University of Nebraska Medical Center
College of Pharmacy
600 South 42nd Street
Omaha, NE 68198-6000
Phone: (800) 626-8431 or (402) 559-4333
Fax: (402) 559-5060
E-mail: mjramire@unmc.edu
Web site: www.unmc.edu/pharmacy/

New Jersey

Rutgers, The State University of New Jersey
Ernest Mario School of Pharmacy
160 Frelinghuysen Road
Piscataway, NJ 08854-8020
Phone: (732) 445-2675
Fax: (732) 445-5767
E-mail: jcolaiz@rci.rutgers.edu
Web site: pharmacy.rutgers.edu/

New Mexico

University of New Mexico
Health Sciences Center
College of Pharmacy
Albuquerque, NM 87131-5691
Phone: (505) 272-2461
Fax: (505) 277-6749
E-mail: wmhadley@unm.edu
Web site: hsc.unm.edu/pharmacy/

New York

Long Island University
The Arnold and Marie Schwartz College of Pharmacy and Health Sciences
75 DeKalb Avenue at University Plaza
Brooklyn, NY 11201-5497
Phone: (718) 488-1004
Fax: (718) 488-0628
E-mail: admissions@brooklyn.liu.edu
Web site: www.liu.edu/cwis/pharmacy/pharmacy.html

St. John's University
College of Pharmacy and Allied Health Professions
8000 Utopia Parkway
Jamaica, NY 11439
Phone: (888) 9ST-JOHNS
Fax: (718) 990-1871
Web site: www.stjohns.edu/pls/portal30/
sjudev.school.pharmacy

State University of New York at Buffalo
School of Pharmacy
C126 Cooke–Hochstetter Complex
Box 601200
Buffalo, NY 14260-1200
Phone: (716) 645-2823
Fax: (716) 645-3688
Web site: wings.buffalo.edu/academic/department/
pharmacy
(PCAT REQUIRED)

Union University
Albany College of Pharmacy
106 New Scotland Avenue
Albany, NY 12208
Phone: (518) 445-7200
Fax: (518) 445-7202
Web site: www.acp.edu/home.php

North Carolina

University of North Carolina at Chapel Hill
School of Pharmacy
CB #7360 Beard Hall
Chapel Hill, NC 27599-7360
Phone: (919) 966-1121
Fax: (919) 966-6919
Web site: www.pharmacy.unc.edu/index.html
(PCAT REQUIRED)

Campbell University
School of Pharmacy
P.O. Box 488
Buies Creek, NC 27506
Phone: (910) 893-1685 or (800) 334-4111, Ext. 1690
Fax: (910) 893-1697
Web site: www.campbell.edu/pharmacy/
(PCAT REQUIRED)

North Dakota

North Dakota State University
College of Pharmacy
Sudro Hall, Room 123
North University Drive & 12 Avenue
Fargo, ND 58105
Phone: (701) 231-6259
Fax: (701) 231-7606
E-mail: Agnes.Harrington@ndsu.nodak.edu
Web site: www.ndsu.edu/ndsu/academic/factsheets/
pharm/pharmacy.shtml
(PCAT REQUIRED)

Ohio

Ohio Northern University
Rudolph H. Raabe College of Pharmacy
Ada, OH 45810
Phone: (419) 772-2275
Fax: (419) 772-2720
Web site: www.onu.edu/Pharmacy

The Ohio State University
College of Pharmacy
217 Parke Hall
500 West 12th Avenue
Columbus, OH 43210-1291
Phone: (614) 292-2266
Fax: (614) 292-2588
Web site: www.pharmacy.ohio-state.edu
(PCAT REQUIRED)

University of Cincinnati-Medical Center
College of Pharmacy
P.O. Box 670004
Cincinnati, OH 45267-0004
Phone: (513) 558-3784
Fax: (513) 558-4372
Web site: vontz.uc.edu/ucfacts.htm

University of Toledo
College of Pharmacy
2801 West Bancroft Street
Toledo, OH 43606
Phone: (419) 530-1904
Fax: (419) 530-1994
E-mail: info@utpharmacy.org
Web site: www.utpharmacy.org/

Oklahoma

Southwestern Oklahoma State University
School of Pharmacy
100 Campus Drive
Weatherford, OK 73096
Phone: (580) 774-3105
Fax: (580) 774-7020
E-mail: Bergmad@SWOSU.edu
Web site: www.swosu.edu/depts/pharmacy
(PCAT REQUIRED)

University of Oklahoma
College of Pharmacy
1110 North Stonewall
P.O. Box 26901
Oklahoma City, OK 73190-5040
Phone: (405) 271-6484
Fax: (405) 271-3830
Web site: www.cpb.uokhsc.edu/
(PCAT REQUIRED)

Oregon

Oregon State University
College of Pharmacy
203 Pharmacy Building
Corvallis, OR 97331-3507
Phone: (541) 737-3424
Fax: (541) 737-3999
Web site: www.orst.edu/dept/cop

Pennsylvania

Duquesne University
Mylan School of Pharmacy
Bayer Learning Center
Pittsburgh, PA 15282
Phone: (412) 396-6380
Fax: (412) 396-5130
Web site: www.pharmacy.duq.edu
(PCAT REQUIRED)

Philadelphia College of Pharmacy
University of the Sciences in Philadelphia
600 South 43rd Street
Philadelphia, PA 19104-4495
Phone: (215) 596-8870
Fax: (215) 596-8977
Web site: www.usip.edu/pcp/

Temple University of the Commonwealth
System of Higher Education
School of Pharmacy
3307 North Broad Street
Philadelphia, PA 19140
Phone: (215) 707-4990
Fax: (215) 707-3678
Web site: www.temple.edu/pharmacy

University of Pittsburgh
School of Pharmacy
1104 Salk Hall
Pittsburgh, PA 15261-1911
Phone: (412) 648-8579
Fax: (412) 648-1086
Web site: www.pharmacy.pitt.edu

Nesbitt School of Pharmacy
Wilkes University
School of Science and Engineering
Box 111
Wilkes-Barre, PA 18766
Phone: (570) 408-4280 or (800)-WILKESU, Ext. 4823
Fax: (570) 408-7828
E-mail: pharm@wilkes.edu
Web site: pharmacy.wilkes.edu
(PCAT RECOMMENDED)

LECOM School of Pharmacy
Lake Erie College of Osteopathic Medicine
1858 West Grandview Boulevard
Erie, Pennsylvania 16509-1025
Phone: (814) 866-6641
Fax: (814) 866-8450
E-mail: pharmacy@lecom.edu
Web site: www.lecom.edu/pharmacy

Puerto Rico

University of Puerto Rico
School of Pharmacy
P.O. Box 365067, University Station
Rio Piedras, PR 00936-5067
Phone: (787) 758-2525, Ext. 5400
Fax: (787) 751-5680
Web site: www.rcm.upr.clu.edu/academics.html
(PCAT REQUIRED)

Rhode Island

University of Rhode Island
College of Pharmacy
Fogarty Hall
41 Lower College Road
Kingston, RI 02881-0809
Phone: (401) 874-5842
Fax: (401) 874-2181
E-mail: pharmcol@etal.uri.edu
Web site: www.uri.edu/pharm/

South Carolina

College of Pharmacy
Medical University of South Carolina
280 Calhoun Street
P.O. Box 250141
Charleston, SC 29425-2301
Phone: (843) 792-3115
Fax: (843) 792-9081
Web site: www.musc.edu/pharmacy/

College of Pharmacy
University of South Carolina
Columbia, SC 29208
Phone: (803) 777-4151
Fax: (803) 777-2775
Web site: www.pharm.sc.edu
(PCAT REQUIRED)

South Dakota

College of Pharmacy
South Dakota State University
Box 2202C
Brookings, SD 57007-0099
Phone: (605) 688-6197
Fax: (605) 688-6232
Web site: www3.sdstate.edu/Academics/
CollegeofPharmacy/index.cfm

Tennessee

University of Tennessee
College of Pharmacy
847 Monroe Avenue
Memphis, TN 38163
Phone: (901) 448-6036
Fax: (901) 448-7053
Web site: www.utmem.edu/pharm/pharm.html
(PCAT REQUIRED)

Texas

Texas Southern University
College of Pharmacy and Health Sciences
3100 Cleburne
Houston, TX 77004
Phone: (713) 313-7164
Fax: (713) 313-1091
Web site: www.tsu.edu/pharmacy
(PCAT REQUIRED)

University of Houston
College of Pharmacy
4800 Calhoun Boulevard
Houston, TX 77204-5511
Phone: (713) 743-1300
Fax: (713) 743-1259
Web site: www.pharmacy.uh.edu/
(PCAT REQUIRED)

University of Texas at Austin
College of Pharmacy
1 University Station, A1900
Austin, TX 78712-0120
Phone: (512) 471-1737
Fax: (512) 471-8783
E-mail: pharmacy@www.utexas.edu
Web site: www.utexas.edu/pharmacy
(PCAT REQUIRED)

Texas Tech University Health Science Center
School of Pharmacy
1300 South Coulter Street
Amarillo, TX 79106
Phone: (806) 354-5463
Fax: (806) 354-4017
E-mail: arthur@cortex.ama.ttuhsc.edu
Web site: ismo.ama.ttuhsc.edu/ExternalHome/
(PCAT REQUIRED)

Utah

University of Utah
College of Pharmacy
30 South 2000 East, Room 201
Salt Lake City, UT 84112-5820
Phone: (801) 581-6731
Fax: (801) 581-3716
E-mail: jmauger@deans.pharm.utah.edu
Web site: www.pharmacy.utah.edu

Virginia

School of Pharmacy
Hampton University
Hampton, VA 23668
Phone: (757) 727-5071
Fax: (757) 727-5840
Web site: www.hamptonu.edu/Pharm/Index.htm
(PCAT REQUIRED)

Virginia Commonwealth University
School of Pharmacy/VCU
MCV Campus—Box 980581
410 North 12th Street
Richmond, VA 23298-0581
Phone: (804) 828-3000
Fax: (804) 828-7436
Web site: www.pharmacy.vcu.edu
(PCAT STRONGLY RECOMMENDED)

Shenandoah University
Bernard J. Dunn School of Pharmacy
1460 University Drive
Winchester, VA 22601
Phone: (540) 665-1282 or (888) 420-7877
Fax: (540) 665-1283
Web site: pharmacy.su.edu
(PCAT REQUIRED)

Washington

University of Washington
School of Pharmacy
Box 357631
H-364 Health Science Building
Seattle, WA 98195-7631
Phone: (206) 543-2030
Fax: (206) 685-9297
E-mail: sidnels@u.washington.edu
Web site: depts.washington.edu/pha/
(PCAT REQUIRED)

Washington State University
College of Pharmacy
105 Wegner Hall
P.O. Box 646510
Pullman, WA 99164-6510
Phone: (509) 335-8664
Fax: (509) 335-0162
Web site: www.pharmacy.wsu.edu

West Virginia

West Virginia University
Health Sciences Center
School of Pharmacy
WVU HSC 1136 HSN
P.O. Box 9500
Morgantown, WV 26506-9500
Phone: (304) 293-5101
Fax: (304) 293-5483
Web site: www.hsc.wvu.edu/sop/
(PCAT REQUIRED)

Wisconsin

University of Wisconsin-Madison
School of Pharmacy
777 Highland Avenue
Madison, WI 53705-2222
Phone: (608) 262-1416
Fax: (608) 262-3397
Web site: www.pharmacy.wisc.edu
(PCAT REQUIRED)

Wyoming

University of Wyoming
School of Pharmacy
P.O. Box 3375
Laramie, WY 82071-3375
Phone: (307) 766-6120
Fax: (307) 766-2953
Web site: www.uwyo.edu/pharmacy
(PCAT REQUIRED)

STATE BOARDS OF PHARMACY

Alabama State Board of Pharmacy
1 Perimeter Park South, Suite 425 South
Birmingham, AL 35243
Phone: (205) 967-0130
Fax: (205) 967-1009
Web site: www.albop.com

Alaska Board of Pharmacy
P.O. Box 110806
Juneau, AK 99811-0806
Phone: (907) 465-2589
Fax: (907) 465-2974
Web site: www.dced.state.ak.us/occ/ppha.htm

Arizona State Board of Pharmacy
4425 W. Olive Avenue, Suite 140
Glendale, AZ 85302
Phone: (623) 463-2727
Fax: (623) 934-0583
Web site: www.pharmacy.state.az.us

Arkansas State Board of Pharmacy
101 East Capitol, Suite 218
Little Rock, AR 72201
Phone: (501) 682-0190
Fax: (501) 682-0195
Web site: www.state.ar.us/asbp

California Board of Pharmacy
400 R Street, Suite 4070
Sacramento, CA 95814
Phone: (916) 445-5014
Fax: (916) 327-6308
Web site: www.pharmacy.ca.gov/

Colorado State Board of Pharmacy
1560 Broadway, Suite 1310
Denver, CO 80202
Phone: (303) 894-7750
Fax: (303) 894-7764
Web site: www.dora.state.co.us/pharmacy

Connecticut Pharmacy Commission
165 Capitol Avenue, Room 147
Hartford, CT 06106
Phone: (860) 713-6065
Fax: (860) 713-7242
Web site: www.ctdrugcontrol.com/rxcommision.htm

Delaware State Board of Pharmacy
Jesse S. Cooper Building, Room 205
PO Box 637
Dover, DE 19903
Phone: (302) 739-4798
Fax: (302) 739-3071
Web site: www.professionallicensing.state.de.us/boards/pharmacy/index

District of Columbia Board of Pharmacy
825 North Capitol Street NE, 2nd Floor
Washington, D.C. 20002
Phone: (202) 442-4776
Fax: (202) 442-9431
Web site: dchealth.dc.gov/prof_license/services/boards_main.asp

Florida Board of Pharmacy
NorthWood Center
4052 Bald Cypress Way, Bin #CO4
Tallahassee, FL 32399-3254
Phone: (850) 245-4292
Fax: (850) 413-6982
Web site: www.doh.state.fl.us/mqd

Georgia State Board of Pharmacy
237 Coliseum Drive
Macon, GA 31217-3858
Phone: (478) 207-1686
Fax: (478) 207-1699
Web site: www.sos.state.ga.us/plb/pharmacy/

Hawaii State Board of Pharmacy
P.O. Box 3469
Honolulu, HI 96801
Phone: (808) 586-2694
Web site: www.hawaii.gov/dcca/pvl/areas-pharmacy.html

Idaho Board of Pharmacy
3380 Americana Terrace, Suite 320
P.O. Box 83720
Boise, ID 83720-0067
Phone: (208) 334-2356
Fax: (208) 334-3536
Web site: www.state.id.us/bop

Illinois State Board of Pharmacy
Illinois Department of Professional Regulation
320 West Washington, 3rd Floor
Springfield, IL 62786
Phone: (217) 785-0800
Fax: (312) 814-4500 (Chicago office)
Web site: www.dpr.state.il.us/WHO/phar.asp

Indiana Board of Pharmacy
402 West Washington Street, Room 041
Indianapolis, IN 46204-2739
Phone: (317) 232-2960
Fax: (317) 233-4236
Web site: www.in.gov/hpb/boards/isbp/

Iowa Board of Pharmacy Examiners
400 SW Eighth Street, Suite E
Des Moines, IA 50309-4688
Phone: (515) 281-5944
Fax: (515) 281-4609
Web site: www.state.ia.us/ibpe

Kansas State Board of Pharmacy
Landon State Office Building
900 SW Jackson Street, Room 513
Topeka, KS 66612-1231
Phone: (785) 296-4056 or 888-RXBOARD
Fax: (785) 296-8420
Web site: www.accesskansas.org/pharmacy

Kentucky Board of Pharmacy
23 Millcreek Park
Frankfort, KY 40601-9230
Phone: (502) 573-1580
Fax: (502) 573-1582
Web site: www.state.ky.us/boards/pharmacy

Louisiana Board of Pharmacy
5615 Corporate Boulevard, Suite 8E
Baton Rouge, LA 70808-2537
Phone: (225) 925-6496
Fax: (225) 925-6499
Web site: www.labp.com

Maine Commission on Pharmacy
Department of Professional & Financial Regulation,
Office of Licensing & Registration
35 State House Station
Augusta, ME 04333-0035
Phone: (207) 624-8620
Fax: (207) 624-8637
E-mail: kelly.l.mclaughlin@state.me.us
Web site: www.state.me.us/pfr/olr/categories/cat30.htm

Maryland Board of Pharmacy
4201 Patterson Avenue
Baltimore, MD 21215-2299
Phone: (410) 764-4755
Fax: (410) 358-6207
E-mail: MDBOP@DHMH.STATE.MD.US
Web site: www.dhmh.state.md.us/pharmacyboard/

Massachusetts Board of Registration in Pharmacy
239 Causeway Street, Suite 500
Boston, MA 02114
Phone: (617) 727-9953
Fax: (617) 727-2197
Web site: www.state.ma.us/reg/boards/ph

Michigan Board of Pharmacy
P.O. Box 30018
Lansing, MI 48909-8170
Phone: (517) 335-0918
Fax: (517) 373-2179
Web site: michigan.gov/cis/0,1607,7-154-
10568_17671_17688-42779--,00.html

Minnesota Board of Pharmacy
2829 University Avenue SE, Suite 530
Minneapolis, MN 55414-3251
Phone: (612) 617-2201
Fax: (612) 617-2212
Web site: www.phcybrd.state.mn.us

Mississippi Board of Pharmacy
625 North State Street
Jackson, MS 39202
Phone: (601) 354-6750
Fax: (601) 354-6071
Web site: www.mbp.state.ms.us

Missouri State Board of Pharmacy
P.O. Box 625
Jefferson City, MO 65102
Phone: (573) 751-0091
Fax: (573) 526-3464
Web site: www.ecodev.state.mo.us/pr/pharmacy

Montana Board of Pharmacy
PO Box 200513
Helena, MT 59620-0513
Phone: (406) 841-2356
Fax: (406) 841-2343
Web site: www.discoveringmontana.com/dii/bsd/
license/bsd_boards/pha_board/board_page.htm

Nebraska Bureau of Examining Boards
P.O. Box 95007
Lincoln, NE 68509-5007
Phone: (402) 471-2118
Web site: www.hhs.state.ne.us

Nevada State Board of Pharmacy
555 Double Eagle Court, Suite 1100
Reno, NV 89511-8991
Phone: (775) 850-1440 or (800) 364-2081
Fax: (775) 850-1444
Web site: www.state.nv.us/pharmacy

New Hampshire Board of Pharmacy
57 Regional Drive
Concord, NH 03301-8518
Phone: (603) 271-2350
Fax: (603) 271-2856
Web site: www.state.nh.us/pharmacy/

New Jersey Board of Pharmacy
P.O. Box 45013
Newark, NJ 07101
Phone: (800) 242-5846
Fax: (973) 648-3355
Web site: www.state.nj.us/lps/ca/brief/pharm.htm

New Mexico Board of Pharmacy
University Towers
1650 University Boulevard NE, Suite 400B
Albuquerque, NM 87102
Phone: (800) 565-9102 or (505) 841-9102
Fax: (505) 841-9113
Web site: www.state.nm.us/pharmacy

New York Board of Pharmacy
NYS Education Department
Division of Professional Licensing Services
State Education Building, 2nd Floor
Albany, NY 12234-1000
Phone: (518) 474-3848
Fax: (518) 473-6995
Web site: www.nysed.gov/prof/pharm.htm

North Carolina Board of Pharmacy
P.O. Box 459
Carrboro, NC 27510-0459
Phone: (919) 942-4454
Fax: (919) 967-5757
Web site: www.ncbop.org

North Dakota Board of Pharmacy
P.O. Box 1354
Bismarck, ND 58502-1354
Phone: (701) 328-9535
Fax: (701) 258-9312
Web site: www.nodakpharmacy.com

Ohio State Board of Pharmacy
77 South High Street, Room 1702
Columbus, OH 43215-6126
Phone: (614) 466-4143
Fax: (614) 752-4836
Web site: www.state.oh.us/pharmacy/

Oklahoma State Board of Pharmacy
4545 Lincoln Boulevard, Suite 112
Oklahoma City, OK 73105-3488
Phone: (405) 521-3815
Fax: (405) 521-3758
Web site: www.pharmacy.state.ok.us/

Oregon Board of Pharmacy
State Office Building, Suite 425
800 NE Oregon Street #9
Portland, OR 97232
Phone: (503) 731-4032
Fax: (503) 731-4067
Web site: www.pharmacy.state.or.us

Pennsylvania State Board of Pharmacy
P.O. Box 2649
Harrisburg, PA 17105-2649
Phone: (717) 783-7156
Fax: (717) 787-7769
Web site: www.dos.state.pa.us/bpoa/phabd/
mainpage.htm

Puerto Rico Board of Pharmacy
Department of Health, Board of Pharmacy
Call Box 10200
Santurce, PR 00908
Phone: (787) 725-8161

Rhode Island State Board of Pharmacy
3 Capitol Hill, Room 205
Providence, RI 02908
Phone: (401) 222-2837
Fax: (401) 222-2158
Web site: www.healthri.org/hsr/professions/
pharmacy.htm

South Carolina Board of Pharmacy
P.O. Box 11927
Columbia, SC 29211-1927
Phone: (803) 896-4700
Fax: (803) 896-4596
Web site: www.llr.state.sc.us/pol/pharmacy

South Dakota Board of Pharmacy
4305 S. Louise Ave., Suite 104
Sioux Falls, SD 57106
Phone: (605) 362-2737
Fax: (605) 362-2738
Web site: www.state.sd.us/dcr/pharmacy

Tennessee Board of Pharmacy
Davy Crockett Tower
500 James Robertson Parkway, 2nd Floor
Nashville, TN 37243-1149
Phone: (615) 741-2718
Fax: (615) 741-2722
Web site: www.state.tn.us/commerce/pharmacy

Texas State Board of Pharmacy
William P. Hobby Building
Tower 3, Suite 600
333 Guadalupe Street, Box 21
Austin, TX 78701
Phone: (512) 305-8000
Fax: (512) 305-8082
Web site: www.tsbp.state.tx.us

Utah Board of Pharmacy
160 East 300 South
P.O. Box 146741
Salt Lake City, UT 84114-6741
Phone: (801) 530-6628
Fax: (801) 530-6511
Web site: www.dopl.utah.gov/licensing/pharmacy.html

Vermont State Board of Pharmacy
26 Terrace Street, Drawer 09
Montpelier, VT 05609-1106
Phone: (802) 828-2875
Fax: (802) 828-2465
Web site: www.vtprofessionals.org/opr1/pharmacists/

Virginia State Board of Pharmacy
6603 West Broad Street, 5th Floor
Richmond, VA 23230-1712
Phone: (804) 662-9911
Fax: (804) 662-9313
Web site: www.dhp.state.va.us/pharmacy/default.htm

Virgin Island Board of Pharmacy
Roy L. Schneider Hospital
48 Sugar Estate
St. Thomas, VI 00802
Phone: (340) 774-0117
Fax: (340) 777-4001

Washington State Board of Pharmacy
P.O. Box 47863
Olympia, WA 98504-7863
Phone: (360) 236-4825
Fax: (360) 586-4359
Web site: wws2.wa.gov/doh/hpqa-licensing/HPS4/
Pharmacy/default.htm

West Virginia Board of Pharmacy
232 Capitol Street
Charleston, WV 25301
Phone: (304) 558-0558
Fax: (304) 558-0572
Web site: www.wvbop.com/main.htm

Wisconsin Pharmacy Examining Board
State of Wisconsin
Depart. Of Regulation & Licensing
P.O. Box 8935
Madison, WI 53708-8935
Phone: (608) 266-2812
Fax: (608) 261-7083
E-mail: web@drl.state.wi.us
Web site: www.drl.state.us/

Wyoming State Board of Pharmacy
1720 South Poplar Street, Suite 4
Casper, WY 82601
Phone: (307) 234-0294
Fax: (307) 234-7226
Web site: pharmacyboard.state.wy.us

Give Your Admissions Essay An Edge At...

EssayEdge.com

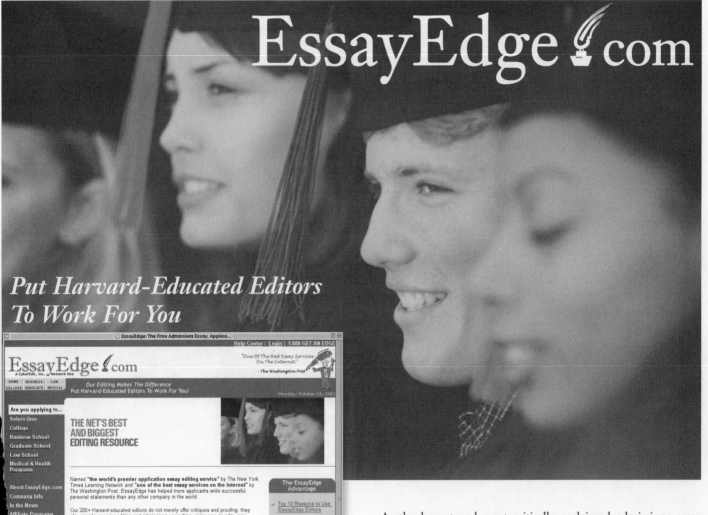

*Put Harvard-Educated Editors
To Work For You*

As the largest and most critically acclaimed admissions essay service, EssayEdge.com has assisted countless college, graduate, business, law, and medical program applicants gain acceptance to their first choice schools. With more than 250 Harvard-educated editors on staff, EssayEdge.com provides superior editing and admissions consulting, giving you an edge over hundreds of applicants with comparable academic credentials.

Visit **www.essayedge.com today,**
and take your admissions essay to a new level.

"One of the Best Essay Services on the Internet"
—The Washington Post

World's Premier Application Essay Editing Service"
—The New York Times Learning Network

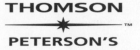

Your everything education destination... the *all-new* Petersons.com

When education is the question, **Petersons.com** is the answer. Log on today and discover what the *all-new* Petersons.com can do for you. Find the ideal college or grad school, take an online practice admission test, or explore financial aid options—all from a name you know and trust, Peterson's.

www.petersons.com

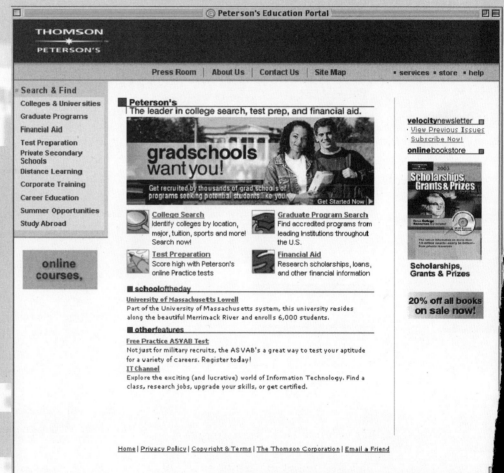

THOMSON
PETERSON'S™